ALSO BY STEPHAN B. POULTER, PhD

The Shame Factor: Heal Your Deepest Fears and Set Yourself Free

The Art of Successful Failure!

Your Ex-Factor: Overcome Heartbreak and Build a Better Life

The Mother Factor: How Your Mother's Emotional Legacy Impacts Your Life

The Father Factor: How Your Father's Legacy Impacts Your Career

Father Your Son: How to Become the Father You've Always Wanted to Be

*Mending the Broken Bough: Restoring the Promise of
the Mother and Daughter Relationship*

T0243858

To all the men who are helping the brotherhood
embrace their modern masculinity journey

MODERN MASCULINITY

A Compassionate Guidebook to Men's Mental Health

STEPHAN B. POULTER, PhD

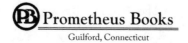

Prometheus Books

Guilford, Connecticut

Ⓟ Prometheus Books

An imprint of Globe Pequot, the trade division of The Rowman & Littlefield
Publishing Group, Inc.
4501 Forbes Blvd., Ste. 200
Lanham, MD 20706
www.rowman.com

Distributed by NATIONAL BOOK NETWORK

British Library Cataloguing in Publication Information Available

Library of Congress Cataloging-in-Publication Data

Names: Poulter, Stephan, author.
Title: Modern masculinity : a compassionate guidebook to men's mental health /
    Stephan B. Poulter, PhD.
Description: Lanham, MD : Prometheus Books, [2024] | Includes bibliographical
    references. | Summary: "Modern Masculinity is a practical guide for men of all ages
    to embrace their on-going process of developing a balanced, compassionate, and
    positive masculinity"—Provided by publisher.
Identifiers: LCCN 2023033070 (print) | LCCN 2023033071 (ebook) |
    ISBN 9781633889422 (paperback) | ISBN 9781633889439 (epub)
Subjects: LCSH: Masculinity. | Men—Psychology. | Men—Mental health.
Classification: LCC BF692.5 .P675 2024 (print) | LCC BF692.5 (ebook) |
    DDC 155.3/32—dc23/eng/20230824
LC record available at https://lccn.loc.gov/2023033070
LC ebook record available at https://lccn.loc.gov/2023033071

♾️™ The paper used in this publication meets the minimum requirements of
American National Standard for Information Sciences—Permanence of Paper for
Printed Library Materials, ANSI/NISO Z39.48-1992

CONTENTS

READER'S NOTE

All the stories, examples, and voices in this book are derived in part from more than forty-five years of personal, professional, research, law enforcement, and life experience. However, the names, places, and other identifying details have been altered to protect the privacy and anonymity of these individuals. Any similarities between the names and stories of the individuals and families described in this book and other individuals are purely coincidental.

FOREWORD

As I write this, I'm watching the NBA playoffs, hoping to see a good basketball game. It matters little to me who wins and who loses, for I've got no skin in the game at all, but I do enjoy a good contest. I no longer cheer for any specific players or teams nor can I envision myself performing any of the athletic feats of these young men today, though I once did, and I certainly can't fathom dressing in their fashion trends! What I can connect to now, however, are the concerns of the mental wellness of a certain NBA phenom who can jump out of the gym, leaving the crowd amazed, on the edges of their seats, while he simultaneously indulges in gunplay at clubs, in cars, and near NBA facilities. His actions appear to confuse family, friends, enemies, and casual observers. Some ask, "Wasn't he just exercising his Second Amendment right?" Others say, "Doesn't he realize what he has to lose?" And yet others wonder if he knows he is a role model.

A local police department received a call a few days ago that a man's brother had been missing since January. Six months later, the missing man's vehicle was found in the parking lot of a major retailer. Among the heap of trash and what looked to be the man's only personal items sat his decomposed body. I was told that the deceased had struggled with addiction and loneliness for some time. The irony of the find was that the vehicle was parked directly across the street from the police department! No one reported the man missing for six months, and no officer suspected anything amiss, though the vehicle sat there for almost 170 days.

We've got to be honest. Men around the world have been struggling with mental, physical, psychological, financial, and spiritual health and well-being for a long time, and a good number of us have done everything we can to look the other way.

I recognized this elephant in the room in 2011 when I lost my close friend to addiction. He'd been struggling to come to terms with a humiliating marriage wherein he was relegated to participating in threesomes with his wife or watching her engage in sexual acts with other men. He was a father to a young toddler, but he wasn't happy. The son he doted on during infancy was later diagnosed with autism. It was heartbreaking for him and just too much to process for his wife. With little to no support, they both sought pleasurable distractions to numb their pain. I'll never forget that 2:00 a.m. phone call when he told me he was doing well, and he sounded relaxed and optimistic. We talked for close to two hours that early morning. Six hours later, his cousin called to tell me his wife found him dead with a needle in his arm and my number queued up on his phone.

This gave birth to the Barbershop Group and my eventual meeting and subsequent work with Dr. Poulter and so many other helpers and healers around the world. Silent suffering isn't "manly," though we've done it time and time again. Many of us learned it from our fathers, grandfathers, and other men in our lives. Some of us learned it from mothers who were focused on survival and who thought that being a good mother meant teaching sons to be the hard, cold, calculative men they tried to love. We have amassed a harrowing number of traumatic experiences that we struggled to cope with for years, only for them to resurface in our marriages, workplaces, schools, and various relationships.

Whether you're a phenomenal athlete or blue-collar construction laborer, your mind and body matter, your thoughts matter, your health matters. If men don't get help—and soon—we will set ourselves on fire, and our loved ones may be resigned to watch us burn.

There is a choice, however. It is my hope that you will earnestly delve into the words found within this comprehensive text. Almost every aspect of men's lives have been covered herein. It won't be an easy read, and it won't provide a fleeting high. I promise you that if you take the time to dissect this alone or, hopefully, with other men and possibly even a therapist, you will begin to experience new life.

Until we meet, love you and love your people more,

—Charles Catchings, founder, the Barbershop Group

FOREWORD

My sons just left for a Yankees–Dodgers game with their father, and I'm at home with my husband and my two spoiled dogs, both male. I've spent a better part of my adult life surrounded by males, and I like it that way. I didn't know the gender of my kids before they were born, but my standing joke is "God knew I wanted boys." I grew up with a sister and two brothers who were much younger than my sister and me, so it felt like I was able to "practice" with them.

Parenthood is full of challenges, but one consistent goal in my eighteen-year parenting journey has been to remind both my sons every day that they are important, strong, capable, and not inherently faulty people. For as long as I can remember, the narrative with boys has been that—in comparison to girls—they are "immature," "behind," "rowdy," "rough," and "detached." When I applied for preschool for my oldest son, several mothers told me to hold him back because of his summer birthday, a common practice called "redshirting." They assured me that he'd be too young once schooling moved along. I followed my instincts and enrolled him, and at no point in his now-finished high school career did he prove to be unready.

Being a mother, wife, and daughter who cherishes the men in her life, hearing this negative notion that men are "toxic" or "aggressive" feels misdirected on every level. Men have played an enormous part in my success as an adult. I feel a duty to defend the notion of masculinity since it's not a negative thing but a necessary part of modern society. Men's mental health matters.

Our society has placed men and women in two different categories when it comes to emotional learning and intelligence. It's held that one side—the female—works on it and the other side—the male—does not. But as human beings, we all strive to be better versions of ourselves, and it's time to include men in this dialogue.

The day my oldest son came to me during the school lockdowns of 2020 and said, "Mom, I think I need someone to talk to who isn't you," I felt a wave of emotion. But I wasn't only sad about the aloneness that I knew he felt, I was also proud of him. He was able to move past the cultural expectations of just "sucking it up" and "getting on with it." It was then that our family was introduced to Dr. Poulter, and he's been a beacon of healthy masculinity for our family ever since.

We women who love men want to help them. If we could heal what's causing them pain, we would. But we can't unless there's a bridge we can use to bring the two sides together. We females who have fathers, uncles, brothers, sons, neighbors, husbands, and other men in our lives and who long for a guide to male mental health now have that: a book to keep on our shelves that can help us do that.

Putting in the work it takes to get ourselves to a healthy place is not always easy, but it's worth it. This book offers a step-by-step guide to a more stable life and a full emotional bank account.

All men deserve to be seen and understood. We women see you, we care, and we need you.

—Angela DiGaetano, mother, wife, and supporter of men

ACKNOWLEDGMENTS

I want to acknowledge all the men in my life (past and present) who have pushed me to be a better man. I want to acknowledge the integral woman in my life who has pushed me to be my best self: my wife Miriam.

Miriam has been telling me for years that I need to address the father-son masculine crisis, as has my fellow therapist Charles Catchings. Sincere thanks to Jake Bonar for taking my phone calls and believing in our process. These three people were incredibly supportive and compassionate. Thank you to all the mothers, wives, and daughters who have expressed concern for their men and worried about them. Thank you to my family near and far who believe in me and don't always understand me.

There are too many names to list, but I need to mention a few who have been instrumental in my growth over the last twenty-five years: Barry Weichman, Jim Myerson, Brad Jenkins, Chris L. Casey, Carter Felts, my two sons, my two daughters, my clients, my three beagles, and the brotherhood.

INTRODUCTION

Men's Health and Masculinity: Why It Matters

True masculinity is showing love, showing compassion, showing all these things that are traditionally not spoken of as masculinity, and that scares some people.—Brandon Bures

I am not sure how or when the topic of being a man evolved within me, but my best guess is that it started around age twelve on the black asphalt playground in La Crescenta, California. It was a fall Saturday afternoon and all the kids in the neighborhood would play tackle football. (I know it was stupid, but we were young, fearless boys.) A kid named Bruce brought his five-horsepower gas-powered minibike that day and was riding it around on the field. You know what happened?

Bruce accidentally ran into me as I was trying to jump out of the way. Instead, I landed on his handlebars and we both crashed. After that introduction, Bruce and I became lifelong friends and brothers. Both our mothers had the same first name, Charlotte, which freaked us out. Our moms—Charlotte 1 and 2—were tough-minded women who had little tolerance for teenaged-boy shenanigans, such as minibikes and tackle football on cement. Another interesting fact was that our fathers were emotionally absent, as were most of the thirty to forty boys playing that day on the playground. I wondered sometimes where my buddies' dads were. We lived in nice homes, we all had fathers, but they weren't watching us grow up.

Fast forward to spring 2022, when Bruce calls me and tells me he has a progressive cancer diagnosis, and it isn't good. Bruce says,

Poult [my childhood nick name], you are a great dad. Be a good dad to my sons. They need to be healthy, loving, caring, kind, and compassionate men. I have a lot of anger about my childhood. I haven't been very good at telling the boys or my wife how much I love them. I am not good at that emotional feeling stuff like you, but I am going to change it while I have time. I showed them my love by working and creating a company. I need to get things right emotionally, psychologically, and spiritually, Poult. I have never gotten over my resentment toward my mom for being so hard on me about my dad's absence. My parents divorced, my dad wasn't around very much, and I didn't want that for my boys.

I was at a loss for words. I had never heard Bruce describe or speak so clearly about his feelings, thoughts, and hopes. Bruce is the super-accomplished guy we all want to be: he has three wonderful young-adult sons, a loving wife, and wealth. This was a painful reminder that our inner life is equally, if not more important than our careers, sports, money, and prestige. My voice was shaky as I tried to say something wise and caring. All I could say was, "Bruce, I am so sorry, and we will get through this." We hung up after telling each other how we loved each other—that was also not typical. That afternoon was an emotional blur. I canceled the rest of my appointments for that day and the next. I couldn't stop thinking how guys like Bruce seem bulletproof due to unresolved anger, fatherlessness, shame, and despair. There are men who look seemingly indestructible yet experience disappointment, illness, heartbreak, despair, trauma, and death. Men need their complete health, not just the su-perficial appearance of "looking good."

Among the things I learned about men professionally and personally over the years is the simple truth that we can foster a balanced life outwardly and inwardly, even in this enlightened age of technology. The use of smartphones and scientific discoveries abound about everything leaving men in emotional straitjackets. Teenagers, twentysomethings, middle-aged and old men un-knowingly and unconsciously attempt to conform to being a "man" without the complete masculine "toolbox" in hand. Our families, colleagues, and friends wonder what's going on with this male revolution.

One thing is a glaring warning sign: avoiding our psychology and physical health can't be dismissed, minimized, or trivialized any longer. Our partners, sisters, daughters—and even younger men themselves—are demanding an-swers and change. Men are now faced with looking within for answers. This requires us to drop the false bravado that our physical health, relationships, emotions, and self-doubts are somehow self-indulgent accesso-ries, rather than lifesaving requirements for navigating our lives.

Masculine fact: Men aren't psychologically bulletproof—life demands our attention.

The complete 360-degree picture of your life will get your attention eventually. It can come in as many forms and ways as there are men living, and I guarantee that the bill for neglect always comes due. This is a universal truth regardless of culture or religious leanings: the bill comes due. Bruce was fully aware that he had unresolved emotional issues to address. Men know that "things" under the hoods of their masculine engines are in need of a major 60,000-mile tune-up. Men (this includes me) try to drive their lives forward without access to our inner self—physically, emotionally, relationally, and personally. It's not due to irresponsibility or failing to be good providers but rather not knowing how to access or develop a healthy male image and resolve our shame and guilt. Men want to feel better and be better—it's our true nature.

A few months later, I had a therapy session with a young man whom I have known for several years. Scott was seventeen, a high school junior, extremely bright, athletically talented, emotionally guarded (typical teenage boy—man of few words), insightful, and wise beyond his years. We were on the topic of his "friend group" and group text messaging when Scott tells me that he is always the "nice" and "understanding" one among the guys. The kindness isn't returned, and in fact he is frequently mocked by his buddies for it. I asked Scott what bothers him about his friends. Scott told me, "I am not the tough guy or the muscle dude or the self-centered woman chaser. I am nice but it seems no one likes 'nice.' The guys think I am too accepting but I am not going to start a fight to prove I am a man. I am not a man since I will not be an asshole or rude to girls! That means I am not their kind of man. I guess it doesn't bother me that people would think that about me."

Scott further explained that he struggles with trying to conform to his peer group's pressure to be a "cool" guy. Scott doesn't like to drink, vape nicotine, nor verbally or cyberbully others: *"I guess I am not a man. I am okay with that."*

Scott and I talked further about why being kind, emotionally aware, and not physically or emotionally abusive was what men need to be. Scott looked at me and said, "Then being a masculine guy is really being kind? Hmm . . . that's not at my school." Leaning forward with excitement in my voice, "That's it, Scott. Kindness encompasses everything men of any age want—among many other things—and need." When he was nine, Scott lost his father to bone cancer. Beyond their ages, both Bruce and Scott are seemingly different, but are they? The cement wall of denial by men of their emotional and mental health needs isn't an issue that is going away on its own.

THE STATE OF MEN

Let's shift gears for a moment and discuss the quote at the beginning of the chapter, the new masculinity of compassion and kindness, which is an excellent jumping-off point into one of the hottest topics of the day: *men's health and masculinity!* Rarely does a week go by in recent years without a disturbing, heartbreaking news story about an exploitive secretive sexual affair between a male boss and his female subordinate, or sexual abuse in an athletic setting by a coach with his female players, or some type of chronic male sexual advances toward his female or male colleagues. The ongoing storyline of male "entitlement" and "recklessness" has the majority of men cringing. Knowing and witnessing the all-too-common exploits by the worldwide brotherhood of men is troubling. There is a sense of helplessness and disgust floating in the male ether of masculinity.

Younger men (younger than thirty-five) want to stop suppressing, denying, and avoiding their inner self for the sake of looking "good enough" to the guys at the gym, the country club, or at work. Older men (older than thirty-five) want to feel physically, emotionally, relationally, and personally fulfilled. This desire is no longer a luxury but a necessity for longevity. What is currently transpiring within the all-too-familiar masculine definition of success and being a "rugged man" is a poisonous element currently described as "toxic masculinity." The word "toxic," as we are going to use it in our discussion, is as follows: the reckless, abusive power position a man takes with others without regard for his actions and self-absorbed behavior. The toxic man is the dark side of the male masculine model. This type of masculinity is blowing up across every walk of life and at all socioeconomic levels. The alarming stories of violence and sexual and domestic abuse are no longer being tolerated, accepted, or kept secret. What once looked externally successful and masculine often was/is a thin veil of deception covering up for their destructive disregard for colleagues, subordinates, wives, and children. Ultimately these men are a small part of the larger group of fathers and grandfathers who are emotionally showing up, actively involved, and mentoring "civilized" well-balanced young men.

Masculine fact: The abusive man is the dark side of masculinity.

Before going any further, I want to alleviate concerns that I'm blaming or finger-pointing as the flavor-of-the-month other men, or our fathers. Rather, as we begin to drill down into the forbidden, unexplored underside of the masculinity crisis, we are looking for legitimate lasting insights, changes, and resolutions. Second, we are not going to get sidetracked arguing about semantics or political positions. We are taking a different approach to the complex issues men face personally, emotionally, physically, relationally, and financially. The bigger picture of what exactly it means to be a man can no longer be avoided by men. I encourage you to explore and uncover the secret pearls of wisdom and insights buried inside of you.

TWO ELEMENTS OF CHANGE: CURIOSITY AND DESPAIR

Change requires two elements: curiosity and despair. Curiosity is the necessary ingredient for questioning rigid, ingrained beliefs about men by men. Second, being open-minded is required for a three-dimensional view of your mind-body connection, relationship styles, and emotional balance. Finally, despair unfortunately gets our immediate attention and shakes us out from the old way of doing things to consider something new. Despair can be likened to your house being hit by a 200-mile-per-hour tornado and demolishing everything you own and hold dear. All that is left of your life is a pile of rubble and confusion.

Despair combined with shame is your personalized form of psychological terrorism. The force of despair, shame, and panic has no regard for your social standing, wealth, or your accomplishments. Recently, a new client, Ty (age forty-four), came to see me. Two days earlier, his wife of thirteen years had moved out of their family home. Ty was emotionally distraught, having heart palpitations and racing thoughts, and felt lost and didn't know what to do. Ty's marriage had been strained for years. He had refused to go to couples therapy or individual therapy. As I looked at Ty, I could see the fear in his eyes of having "lost" control of his life (or was he gaining control?). It's painful and simultaneously ironic that Ty had argued with his wife about therapy being foolish and a waste of his time.

Unfortunately, Ty was now highly motivated to do anything to save his marriage. It took his wife leaving for him to finally listen and respect her. His wife, Jennifer, had exhausted all her energy fighting with Ty about his lack of concern for her and their three children. Now Ty was desperate to do "anything" to save his marriage and his life.

Change is difficult!

That's why so many men take a pass on making changes until faced with a crisis. The problem with a crisis is that it is out of their control. The circumstances many times present as personal loss (death of loved one), divorce, physical illness (cancer), career setback, or fiscal crisis (loss of net worth).

Over time, psychological resistance to change breeds rigidity of the mind, as William Blake stated more than two hundred years ago. This truism is as applicable today as it was in his lifetime in England during the post–America Revolution era. A curious attitude is necessary, if not mandatory, as we look at the four foundational pillars of your life. Defensiveness about new ideas is a positive sign that you are tapping into the heart of your issues. Superficial change is like spraying perfume on a pig and wondering why it still smells like a pig.

> *The man who never alters his opinion is like standing water, and breeds reptiles of the mind.*—William Blake

For clarity, I am referring to the vast majority of men who are striving to transform inside and out. We aren't going to get off the highway of masculine healing and debate the atrocities of centuries, decades of problematic male behavior. Gentlemen, let's agree that privileged male abuse of years past, the misuse of our social and personal position, is no longer going to be tolerated. We aren't doing an archaeological survey into the past to avoid our responsibility and opportunity to change the present and future. Our purpose is to gain a deeper understanding, practical tools, and solutions for all of us to start using. Oftentimes men want to control the conversation that supports their particular rationalization for "bad" behavior. The result is further exclusion of most men who don't share or engage in negative male choices.

Tolerating and thus accepting another man's differences is one of the features of our new masculinity. This encompasses various sexual orientations, ethnicities, economic levels, career paths, health issues, traumas, cultures, and life experiences. The root of so many problems for men is the old man's template of "be like us." This exclusive, narrow belief system is a fear-based paradigm that fuels racism and prejudice.

Inclusiveness breeds understanding, wisdom, and personal strength.

Gaining insight into the whys and hows of your emotional reactions and mind-body health opens up a whole new world about yourself. Developing our new mental health perspective reveals that we are much more similar than we are different! The emotional and mental acceptance of inclusiveness creates a masculine network of support for you, me, and our world. The fear of differences is a personal issue and topic throughout this book. You wouldn't be reading this book if you weren't looking for deeper fulfillment and contentment in your body, feelings, close relationships, and personal life. Let's try to put aside the knee-jerk reaction of arguing for the sake of "winning" a difference of opinion. It's always a better choice to be kind—which is a sign of strength. A truism of life is that you are always the problem and always the solution. Read that again! Now that the ground rules—we like rules—have been established, let's get back to our discussion.

The majority of men I work with and know don't want to be or be considered "toxic." The term itself implies damaging elements and lethal consequences to those exposed. Cognitive dissonance (the inability to mentally combine two opposing ideas) is a normal response. The uncomfortable but necessary process of peeling back the layers of the onion, also known as emotional scar tissue, can't be emphasized enough. School-age boys, teen boys, young adult males, and older men desperately want to be understood, accepted, and loved. The healing of men starts with men accepting men. It's really that simple.

MEN AND THEIR ROLE MODELS—WHO'S YOURS?

To make use of a road map, you need a destination—we all need one! I don't agree with the adage that a man who lacks a positive role model is doomed to a life of confusion. There is value in understanding the influence our heroes and role models have had on our masculine development. A common complaint by men (and women) is that there aren't positive male role models to follow or emulate. The default reaction by men feeling lost or rudderless is the all-too-common tendency to become the "rugged" male stereotype.

Most men don't like this type of personality and surely don't want to be him. A man attempting to develop a balanced, meaningful life is regarded with suspicion by other men; he is mocked and rejected by the prevailing male peer group. These same men who avoid questioning the status quo of masculinity are in most need of a compassionate masculine relationship. A balanced life is much more than a

Masculinity in the last 150 years has largely been defined by making money and acquiring wealth—this only a small part of a man's life.

positive cash flow every month or large cash reserve. Having insight into one's mental health, bipolar mood swings, anger outbursts, sexual affairs, or compulsive golfing, for example, is a positive masculine influence.

Backstory

The backdrop for the current masculine struggle is necessary to set the stage for how we got here. The most recent shift in manhood started with the Industrial

Revolution in the early 1800s. Masculinity, as a concept, has been in free fall as men search for meaning and purpose. The experience of working away from home caused men to psychologically leave home. The mass migration from farming to industrialization has left men adrift in a sea of confusion about how to be an involved father, husband, and man. Leaving the farm and moving to the city wasn't as easy as many thought. Men were no longer measured by their grit, strength, family name, and courage, but by how much money they earned and their professional achievements.

To fill this male-shaped void, many major cultural images have emerged in the last hundred years. One of the most popular is the silent, rugged male "cowboy" image. A prominent and enduring depiction was that of the "Marlboro Man," who featured in cigarette commercials, riding his horse into the sunset. The irony is that the guy is alone, smoking, and slowly killing himself with emphysema. Another classic cultural icon was the John Wayne type of rugged no-nonsense man.

THE RUGGED COWBOY IMAGE
IS A TIMELESS MALE ICON

When I was fresh out of college, my first job was as a law enforcement officer. Our police academy instructor told us to develop the John Wayne syndrome of being mentally bulletproof from fear, emotionally tall, proud, in great physical shape, and everyone's hero. This was an impossible standard. None of us really understood the implications of being a "badass," but we knew we had to conform to this bigger-than-life image if we wanted to survive.

John Wayne, nicknamed the Duke, was a famous Western cowboy actor from the silent movie era until his death in 1979. Older men (aged sixty and older) were impacted by the famous Rat Pack of Frank Sinatra, Dean Martin, and Sammy Davis Jr. Some other common male icons for boys growing up are Babe Ruth, Joe Namath, Michael Jordan, Derek Jeter, Tiger Woods, Tom Brady, George Clooney, Lebron James, and countless other musicians, athletes, and celebrities who are revered for being rich, famous, and/or gifted. These men personify our nation's image of the "rugged male."

Measuring up to a one-dimensional image is an impossible standard. Every boy had a hero growing up. Who was your hero? Think about why you choose him/her, because there is more significance than you might think. Unconsciously, those who we pick become part of our inner picture of who we are as men.

FILLING THE VOID FOR MEN—
WHO, WHAT, AND WHERE

The male void of masculinity overflows with stories about men behaving poorly with increasing violence toward women and children. We discuss how authentic masculinity comes from deep within, not through physical force. Humble, silent, inward exploration—rather than aggressive outward actions, false bravado, or social status—is a strong force. Men of all ages agree that masculinity has stalled out rather than evolving forward with insight, courage, and kindness.

Today, through a variety of modern technologies of information gathering and sharing (i.e., social media platforms, internet, smartphones, live-streaming videos, etc.), it's a full 360-degree 24/7 exposure of men's behavior. This sheer volume of information and eyewitness accounts

> *Women want men to be responsible, mature, and psychologically balanced.*

is now being communicated around the world within seconds. This is simultaneously alarming and positive. The news media isn't the only source of news or information about men and their questionable behaviors and actions. Women now freely question men's behavior and their secrets. Women independently report to human resources, law enforcement, and the media incidents that, twenty to thirty years ago, were dismissed as "boys being boys." Now these same actions by these adult boys (now fathers, colleagues, coaches, neighbors, Wall Street investors, business owners, etc.) are sexual assaults, nonconsensual sex—date rape—domestic violence, and a host of other illegal activities toward others.

Women now have the courage and platforms to speak up and expose the "old boys club" of favoritism, discrimination, misogyny, and entitlement. "Gentlemen, we have a problem" is a pervasive feeling in corporate boardrooms, on Zoom calls, in classrooms, and on sports teams, starting as young as five all the way to professional levels as well as among women. The corporate and governmental policies exposing domestic violence, abuse, sexual harassment, and violence are ex-

> *The old-school model of masculinity has run out of road. Something new is happening for men.*

cellent starting points. Men ultimately must embrace the masculine shift from rugged aggressiveness to a deeper understanding of their actions, choices, and biases.

The old pattern of concealing "bad" behaviors is no longer possible. Women are now living and working in the same world as men. Accountability and responsibility at home and at work are no longer separate worlds; they are now on the same playing field of life.

> *Our culture has lost a connection to what mature masculinity feels like.*—Connor Beaton

This quote so accurately sums up the widespread disillusionment and backlash against men on the airways, on the internet, and in the media. Wives, mothers, girlfriends, and romantic partners are looking for mature masculine men who seem to be missing in action. Along with this ever-increasing male-shaped vacuum of role confusion, shame, and misunderstanding of men, the biggest surprise is the reaction by men. The sense of hopelessness, denial, and avoidance concerning men's confusion about their masculinity is palpable among men of all walks of life. This is a special time in history. As clinical psychologist for thirty-plus years, my experience is that men tend to have two responses to the current masculinity crisis.

The first is that they believe the stories and yet don't know what steps to take to correct the situation personally with their friends, at school, at work, or at home. The emotional disgust and disappointment in older men is often expressed as: "This is absolutely unacceptable, and change needs to be made." The second response falls at the other end of the spectrum: "What's the big deal? Get over it and stop whining; life isn't fair!"

The first response is usually by younger men ranging from sixteen to thirty-nine years old. The second response is typically by men forty and older. This is a very interesting contrast in responses.

The blatant resistance to change, the denial of the need to update men's Stone Age perspective of life, has its genesis in this rigid belief of how men and the world has always worked. The father factor (your father's spoken and unspoken influence) is another element of the masculinity transformation.

Men of all races, educational backgrounds, and economic levels want to turn the tide against "male bashing" and separate themselves from the cancel-culture movement toward men. These younger men were raised and parented by these older men, but they aren't blindly following or accepting the outdated double-standard that self-centered behavior is okay as long as the perpetrators benefit.

Second, younger men watched and observed their fathers, uncles, and grandfathers making some serious judgment errors in how they have conducted their lives. The younger men want a different type of masculinity, which has all the features of responsibility, secure relationships, courage, strength, and leadership without hurting those in their way. Change is scary and men can't be too "touchy-feely" without ridicule and humiliation by their own brotherhood and close friends.

> *Not until we are lost do we begin to understand ourselves.*—Henry David Thoreau

Another facet of men we explore is the drive to build empire through any means necessary while remaining emotionally disconnected, which leaves millions of men emotionally and psychologically bankrupted. The feelings of emptiness, lack of fulfillment, and shame are some of the common by-products of this modality. Men and the drive for wealth at all costs is under intense scrutiny from all sides and for good reason. Corporate dishonesty at all levels, deliberate exploitation of employees, and personal selfishness isn't tolerated like it once was. The climate of the cutthroat culture of finance isn't socially acceptable by women, who are a major force in the once male-dominated world of business. These all-too-common attitudes have men in a "world of confusion" at home and at work.

Your net worth isn't your self-worth nor a substitution for it.

The relentless pressure to humanize, stop workplace sexual harassment, and accommodate change creates an atmosphere of personal and professional confusion among men. Men are sick of being sick of "bad" behavior in the name of helping the company. Mr. Thoreau, more than 150 years ago, knew that change of beliefs and actions starts only with a deep sense of feeling lost and profoundly disappointed in your role as husband, father, coworker, son, boyfriend, and as a man to other men.

The window of opportunity at hand for change is plausible and attainable for men of any age or circumstance. Regardless of positive or painful life experiences, a man can become the man he has always wanted to be. We are going to explore in detail the four horsemen of masculinity, which are vital for resolving the male crisis with lasting changes within and without.

No one argues about the need for a road map on the 360-degree journey of becoming a complete and fulfilled man. The question that is asked in my office weekly, at happy hour, in gyms, on sports teams, and around the world is, "OK, I agree about being a balanced man but *how*? I have no role models for how to be a man." I patiently remind my clients that they can develop and embrace a balanced, fulfilling life that embodies a healthy male perspective. We address the need for a clear-cut and fully defined masculine road map, which is the purpose of reading and experiencing this book.

CHANGE AND YOUR FOUR HORSEMEN

The horrific saga of Jeffrey Epstein is often discussed as a cautionary tale for men of all races, ages, and economic levels: no man is beyond the hand of justice, regardless of his immense wealth, social power, intelligence, charisma, network of deception, fraud, and lies. This extreme example of self-destruction is opening doors to the possibilities for taking positive paths to succeed as a man. The potential for a compassionate, empathic, enthusiastic, and mentoring masculine man is in stark contrast to the narcissistic maverick man, accountable to no one. The contrast of these two polar opposite masculine models is startling and one of the road markers for shifting our male consciousness out of the Dark Ages and into the present day.

Four foundational aspects of being a man—compassion, empathy, enthusiasm, and mentorship—are the four horsemen. Each man must embrace and master his four horsemen. The character qualities, traits, and psychological understanding of their masculinity empowers boys, young men, and adult men to change their world and the world around them from the inside out. These types of personal shifts have a positive impact today and for generations to come. In each section of the book, I discuss these four major components, which comprise—and are necessary for developing into—a high functioning, emotionally fulfilled, insightful man. The initiative-taking, insightful mental and physical foundation can support any type of building that a young man will create over the course of his life.

> *The true profession of a man is to find his way to himself.*
> —Herman House

The Great Wall of Male Discrimination

Another major factor in the male identity crisis is the social advances that women have been able to accomplish and continue doing.

The "castle of control" for men was fast transforming into a community of equal opportunity. Women began entering the workplace, from which they were once forbidden, based on gender not talent. Male-dominated professions such as finance, law, and medicine could no longer reject women. Long-standing institutions such as the military had to integrate women into their ranks; law enforcement, firefighting, and emergency services all had to accommodate the introduction of women who are equally capable and competent as men. The legal mandate for equal pay was putting the old school on notice that the party was over. These changes toward women's equality—plus many more, including sexual harassment laws and date rape and domestic violence legislation— are making men accountable for their actions.

The male identity crisis has been in the making for years! Society can't cancel masculinity out of boys. Read that again.

Collectively, all of these events have led to the current social momentum of "cancelation culture" surrounding men, being a man, and any type of masculinity, good or bad. The old saying, "Don't throw the baby out with the bathwater," is relevant here. It's imperative for men not to "throw themselves out" because of their confusion, shame, and loss of direction. The quote by Herman House is applicable: men want to find their path to their "best self."

Women are worried about their men!

This discovery many times starts with a tremendous loss, heartbreak, death, or financial ruin. Then the old barriers of denial are immediately wiped out. Despair opens the door to curiosity, and curiosity leads to change. We have all the talents within to embark on the adventure of a lifetime, which is a lifetime journey.

> *I am so pissed off at this cancel culture. Boys are getting unfair treatment and shamed for being a male at school. Young women are misusing their position of whistleblower to crush and devastate the men in their life!*—Alice, age forty-five, mother of two teenage boys

Finally, before beginning our journey into the four corners of masculinity, we need to mention the women in our lives. Women are worried about their men! This may seem counterintuitive based on this discussion but it isn't. We men are connected to the women in our life from the beginning to the end of time. There isn't a grandmother, mother, sister, daughter, auntie, wife, or female colleague who wants their men to disappear into a shame-based life of regret, confusion, and despair, simply for being men. Mothers want their sons, brothers, friends, and husbands to become the men that they have always wanted to be. Women support men. Women see the pain and despair in their eyes and actions. We develop a clear-cut road map for men of all ages, life circumstances, and races to embrace. Gentlemen, we have a plan, a purpose, and a reason to do this. Think about that for a minute.

We present a set of tools—suggestions along with a method for applying them—for men of any age (it's never too late to start on a new path!) to use. Each horseman has a valuable role to play in your life, which is coordinated with the other three horsemen within you.

To map out a course of action and follow it to an end requires courage.—Ralph Waldo Emerson

Having a plan is invaluable for any type of change, small or big. Emerson's timeless quote is absolutely correct: *you* create and follow your map for your personal journey. The funny part of life is that you already have a plan, whether you acknowledge it or not. Making your plan conscious is the first step. The next step is accepting and understanding your manhood as a deliberate choice. Your masculinity, which is part of your core being, requires the same degree of attention as our money market accounts, financial investments, and favorite sports team.

Your life is bigger than your net worth and accomplishments. Your self-worth is something that continually develops throughout your masculine life journey. Self-worth and self-esteem are not stationary; they are a fluid process throughout the valleys and peaks of your life. Many men confuse a strong self-worth as the result of a high net worth. This is a dangerous male myth, which is perpetuated by men, women, and the world at large. Money doesn't make a man; it never has and never will. Money is only part of the overall composite of a man's journey. Financial success is the old standard of measurement for a strong masculinity, which over time turns into a mental health straitjacket.

I know this is a lot of ground to cover. The insightful, empowering pathway for men to experience positive relationships, careers, families, and health usually begins with a personal crisis. For younger men and adolescents, their crisis might come before, during, or after college as an opportunity for sincere introspection. In order to uncover the foundation of our male roots, we need to clean off a lot of debris and gain some honest clarity about our state of being. Many men see this process as threatening and dig their heels into the mud. Many have said to me face-to-face in my office, "Well, that isn't a good option or a productive one for me. I am not into this touchy-feely stuff." My response to this classic knee-jerk response of deflection and denial: "You can do this— it's your manhood."

Men come into my office openly admitting that they just don't know what to do about their life, marriage, kids, career, finances, and resolving their own emptiness. The old achievement markers of success just don't address the deeper longing inside of men. The only two things required to move your life forward is vulnerability and courage. These two psychological virtues are the key to achieving balance and fulfillment in your life. Three questions of the hour:

1. What do men do?
2. How do men do it?
3. How can men survive in a hostile and, at times, man-hating culture?

SUMMARY

The journey to becoming and being a man starts within the hearts of the boys, adolescents, and twentysomethings and continues throughout their lives. Grandfathers and fathers are important men in their lives and will be critical players and untapped sources of information going forward.

We delve into the heart and soul of what it means to be a fulfilled, responsible, healthy, and compassionate man in the twenty-first century. Our deep-dive into heated and volatile issues for men are addressed head-on and include the following:

- Men's emotional needs and mood swings
- Commonly ignored physical health issues
- Mental health and physical health
- Sexual orientation, sexual performance, impotency, sexual abuse, and identity
- Fear of rejection and mothers
- Personal power with or without money
- Male self-acceptance and the ability to form safe and secure relationships with other men
- Narcissism
- Revising financial success as the only standard of manhood
- Removing emotional and psychological straitjackets
- Relationships with your father and mother
- Female anger, codependency, and placating
- Anger management/shame management
- Compassion, empathy, and responsibility
- Removing the male "gag order" regarding shame, sexual abuse, and trauma
- Increasing your emotional, psychological, and relationship IQ
- Body obsession, bodybuilding, your wounded boy, and your father
- The power of forgiveness for you, your parents, your partner, and your siblings
- Crying as a release of control, not masculinity
- Sports, competition, team loyalty, and male bonding
- Therapy and men

- Drinking, womanizing, being a "dude," and your dark side
- The connections between emotional health, relationships, and personal plans
- Emotional roadblocks: shame, imposter syndrome, fear of intimacy, impending doom, fear of authority, and fear of vulnerability

Masculinity develops in the hearts and souls of men, allowing them to experience emotional power and health, physical health and power, relational health and power, and his own plan—his life purpose.

Everyone has a life purpose—everyone!

Feeling emotionally disconnected from themselves and other men and without any tangible means of lasting relief is pushing men inward to resolve this crisis. Men like you can and will answer the many questions and mysteries surrounding modern manhood that no longer need to be buried or avoided. The questions below are both old and current ideas about men, male stereotypes, sex, and relationships. Think about your answers and where you see yourself in terms of evolving, changing, and embracing the next chapter of your life. Let's do a baseline checkup on your perspective of yourself and men with then true or false questions about men.

1. Males express loneliness differently than women. *True or false?*
2. Men crave emotional understanding by their inner circle of male buddies in addition to their romantic partners. *True or false?*
3. Masculinity is an outdated social norm. *True or false?*
4. Compassion, empathy, and acceptance are foundational to a man's mental and physical health, quality of life, and relationship patterns. *True or false?*
5. Sexual harassment of women or men, random sexual partners, and chronic porn viewing are related to the father and son relationship. *True or false?*
6. Male depression and anxiety are signs of immaturity, weakness, and the inability to "man up." *True or false?*
7. Financial success is the primary contribution and role for men in their families and relationships. *True or false?*
8. Romantic heartbreak, divorce, and remarriage are signs of failure and evidence that men can't sustain relationships. *True or false?*
9. Any type of abuse, addiction to drugs, sex, gambling, and personal disappointments are elements of a poor prognosis for change. *True or false?*
10. Sexual intimacy, sexual orientation, sexual compatibility, and sensuality are directly related to a man's understanding of himself and his father. *True or false?*

These questions are designed for you to consider as we leave the safe harbor of "no change" and chart a new course. These psychological and relational concepts are brain teasers, all of which are discussed throughout the book with supporting research and further exploration of the topic at hand: men's health and masculinity and why it matters.

1. Males express loneliness differently than women: *True*. The male expression of loneliness is vastly different from a women's expression of it. Men tend to externalize their anger about feeling lonely and unlovable. Women tend to internalize their sense of loneliness. The experience of isolation and loneliness for extended periods of time is dangerous. Unless this relationship style is addressed, it will develop into paralyzing shame. Another serious side effect of isolation for men of all ages is that it can devolve into aggressive behavior. These behaviors can manifest into forms of self-loathing and self-destructive choices via suicide or homicide. Loneliness is a psychological disconnection from a man's inner sense of self and can create severe mental health issues.

2. Men crave emotional understanding by their inner circle of male buddies in addition to their romantic partners: *True*. Men who report the highest levels of satisfaction, fulfillment, and contentment have strong interpersonal relationships with men. One relationship, marriage, lover, or partner can't fulfill all the needs of a man. Women know and value their girlfriends and their sisterhood of support. Men who develop a close inner circle of male relationships experience the joy and support of their brotherhood. Men do not thrive or maximize their innate potential without the support of other men. No man is an island; he is connected to the generations of men in his family, past and present.

3. Masculinity is an outdated social norm: *False*. The current tide of male bashing is painful to hear, watch, and experience. This period of time in history is the perfect opportunity for a paradigm change for men. The shifting from external ruggedness to internal fortitude, courage, and compassion is necessary for healing families, children, women, and men. The acceptance of personal responsibility for one's actions, decisions, and physical and mental health are some of the ingredients for a fulfilling life.

4. Compassion, empathy, and acceptance are foundational to a man's mental and physical health, quality of life, and relationship patterns: *True*. The new male order is not discarding the enduring qualities of protection, providing, parenting, and career achievement. Rather, the elements of compassion (self-acceptance), empathy (consideration for others), and acceptance (the ability to understand differences) start within. These core

character qualities develop into the positive decisions that men make every day in their relationships, marriages, careers, and personal life. Absent and internally void of these inner qualities, a young man will seek for validation outside of himself. The validation never lasts. This constant need for validation and reassurance is never ending and relentless. Men can develop the emotional bandwidth and secure relationships necessary for embracing themselves and their world. Women know this fact and support their men, sons, and brothers. Women want men to win this battle. The war of the sexes is over; it's now the war to save masculinity!

5. Sexual harassment of women or men, random sexual partners, and chronic porn viewing are related to the father and son relationship: *True*. Men who have had a problematic, strained, abusive, or traumatic father-son relationship typically respond in one of two ways. The first is a reaction to feeling rejected with a sense of competency: *I am capable.* The inner motivation to prove "my old man" wrong is strong and powerful. The other reaction is driven unconsciously by the wounded self-doubting boy within who finds compensatory behaviors, vices, and ultimately addictions to avoid his soul-crushing pain. The maladaptive choices of these boys who become adult men are the causes of self-defeating behaviors and, many times, for horrendous acts toward women, children, and other men. Unresolved trauma between a son and father lasts for generations with unlimited suffering.

6. Male depression and anxiety are signs of immaturity, weakness, and the inability to "man up": *False*. This statement reflects cultural bias against men by other men. Expressing any type of strong emotion other than anger is still too uncomfortable for men of all ages and walks of life to tolerate. Men use merciless humor (humor as a defense mechanism is a classic "man trait") and verbal bullying to prevent other men from talking about deeper issues. The cowboy image of stainless-steel nerves and a soul wrapped in Teflon is still the gold standard for many parts of male culture and world views. Without developing emotional intelligence with sensitivity, a man's physical health, career development, psychological stability, and quality of life is a dead-end street. When feelings, thoughts, and insights are suppressed, they resurface in unhealthy outlets. Emotions are high powered and need positive outlets. The expression of one's feelings is a sign of strength and compassion for self and others. The challenge of "using your words" and not "hitting or hurting others" can be resolved and healed. This is taught in preschool but never past elementary school development in boys who then become fathers, husbands, bosses, and leaders.

7. Financial success is the primary contribution and role for men in their families and relationships: *False*. Using money as a measuring stick for your value, importance in your marriage, family, or male friendships is dangerous. Money isn't evil or bad; it is just not a good master—there is never enough of it. Understanding your attachment to wealth allows other pieces of your personality to emerge. The social pressure and esteem from other men for having sole focus on becoming "rich" is a short-term life plan. Money and its relentless demands (your career) ultimately leave a man morally and emotionally longing for deeper meaning. Men (societal belief) are taught that their fulfillment, peace of mind, and life purpose can be achieved through the accumulation of wealth and all of its benefits. The search for contentment after achieving the "prized" house, career promotion, and so on isn't found in your bank account; it's inside of you. The hyperfocus on wealth creates collateral personal, emotional, and health problems in men. The consequences of neglecting your life are real and painful. One of the keys to a fulfilling life is finding your life purpose; the money will follow.

8. Romantic heartbreak, divorce, and remarriage are signs of failure and evidence that men can't sustain relationships: *False*. Romantic relationships, marriage, and remarriage are important sources of information about who, what, and how you function intimately. The fact that some marriages last only six years while others last sixty years isn't a right or wrong proposition. Rather, the key is understanding that every relationship has both a time limit and value. Knowing that a relationship has run its course in your life requires honesty and courage, along with taking responsibility for your actions and their impact on your partner. "Failure" is not a psychological term and has no value in a person's life. Some of the biggest personal changes occur during and after the end of a relationship. Accepting and addressing repetitive self-defeating behaviors, patterns, and unresolved trauma in your life is the power and value of your relationship history. Men are genetically wired for intimacy, love, and understanding. Avoiding close relationships is a defense mechanism against feeling or being vulnerable. Men crave emotional closeness.

9. Any type of abuse, addiction to drugs, sex, gambling, and personal disappointments are elements of a poor prognosis for change: *False*. The best prognosis for anything in your life is you! Your desire to face and confront self-sabotaging habits, public or private addictions, and the psychological demons and shame that haunt you is all within your grasp. The power of despair and the openness to change via curiosity is a plan that works.

Despair breaks down all the walls surrounding the wounded "tough guy" and "scared self." Curiosity is the opportunity for exposing shame-based beliefs. Unhealed trauma is a loaded gun waiting to be fired at the people in a boy or man's life, literally and figuratively. Our purpose in our masculine dialogue is exposing and healing male shame created by humiliating events in a boy's childhood. Usually, the survivor has a very tough-looking exterior hiding the fearful boy within who longs to be loved and understood. Men need men to embrace their healing journey.

10. Sexual intimacy, sexual orientation, sexual compatibility, and sensuality are directly related to a man's understanding of himself and his father: *True*. Boys imitate, model, and follow their fathers' verbal and nonverbal behaviors, cues, and actions. A young boy by the age of five knows how his father feels about his mother, sister, and women. These seeds of sexuality take root within the young boy. Your sexual identity continues to manifest, influencing consciously and unconsciously and directing your behavior well into adulthood. Sexuality is an essential expression of a man's masculinity. A man's feelings about the issue of sex can be traced back to the father and son relationship.

Part I

BODY MASCULINITY

*The Mind-Body Connection—Physical Health
Is Emotional and Mental Health*

*Ever notice how a guy won't go to the doctor unless his arm
or penis is broken?*—Dr. Jesse N. Mills, MD, founder of the
Men's Health Clinic at University of California at Los Angeles

CHAPTER ONE

LIVING YOUR BEST LIFE PHYSICALLY

How Everything Connects Emotionally and Psychologically to Your Body

Your health is everything, son, and when you have your health, you have everything.—Peter Brett Poulter (1924–2007); my father's sage advice to me

A CAUTIONARY TALE—WHAT IS YOUR BODY SAYING TO YOU?

Roy is a twenty-seven-year-old single male bodybuilder who takes growth hormones intravenously (aka bodybuilding steroids) to maximize his workout results—increased muscle size. Roy has a fast-paced tech sales job that requires him to be at his best emotionally, occupationally, and psychologically. Roy believes that looking "jacked"—muscular—is how men truly judge his masculinity, manhood, business competency, and capabilities. This male stereotype is something we are going to tackle: the appearance of strength doesn't necessarily imply that the man is mentally balanced.

Roy works out six days a week and is a self-described "gym rat." Roy is critical of other guys in the gym: how much they lift, their strength, and muscle size. Roy's father, Mark, also is a gym rat and a bodybuilder in his late sixties. Their father-son relationship has been a deep source of emotional pain for Roy, who, at fifteen, punched his father in the throat when Mark called him a "pussy" for crying after losing his football championship game. Roy made an unspoken pledge to himself that he would never allow anyone to bully or abuse him ever again. Personal oaths, conscious and unconscious, shape our lives (more about this later). Roy's spoken and unspoken oath of self-protection is the foundational glue of his life. Everything Roy does is shaped by his internal self-defense mechanism.

One of his safeguards against being "weak" or a "victim" was to become "jacked physically." Roy's top priority in his life is his physical appearance (he dyes his hair and wears only designer menswear) and his workouts (he trains even when he's sick). Everything else is secondary to his workout regimen including his girlfriend, personal and family relationships, emotions, and feelings. Roy thinks that all the stuff that psychologists discuss is not really important or necessary for a successful life. Roy believes that "psychobabble" distracts from his life force.

Roy's personal mantra, "Get over it," applies to issues in the past that are not relevant today and have no impact on his present day. (I don't believe that Roy truly believes this, although it is what he tells others.) Roy prides himself on not being a "whiner" or a "crybaby" about his life. At the end of this chapter, we return to Roy because his body says a lot about his unexplored psychology, emotional repression, suppression of his childhood trauma, and chronic use of steroids.

YOUR HEALTH IS NOT IN A VACUUM

Our operating theme in part I is that your (young, middle-aged, dad, or older man) body is more than a biological phenomenon operating independently of your day-to-day living. Rather, your body is a complex system interacting with all the conscious and unconscious parts of your life at various levels of immediate awareness. This fact is sometimes good news and sometimes not-so-good news. The question that begs to be asked by any medical, mental health, or psychological professional is: what's going on in your life and body? The answer isn't one-dimensional, but rather three-dimensional, with many factors contributing to the answer.

One of our goals in redefining modern masculinity is starting with your body, a critical part of your mental health and overall quality of life. Without body awareness, it is very difficult to maintain any type of mental health balance and functioning. *It is simply impossible to achieve any significant psychological change, healing, or resolution without body awareness.* Increasing conscious awareness of how our thoughts, feelings, anger, excitement, daily habits, diet, negative self-talk, drinking, sleeping, recreational drug use, relationships, and everyday activities are all interconnected. They impact our heart, blood pressure, liver, back, muscular structure, immune system, brain functioning, and sex drive; the list is endless. Everything in our bodies' functioning—from prenatal, childhood, adolescents, midlife, aging, and our senior years (if we are blessed with a healthy long life)—is connected.

Your body awareness is part of your mental health awareness.

Gentlemen, we can no longer wait for our bodies to signal crisis to take notice. The sense of invincibility is more than a young man's fantasy; rather, it's the delusional foundational cement of the "macho" masculine model. This all-too-common male model is the adolescent belief that you are more powerful than life and will defeat Father Time. No one escapes the natural evolution of life—no one! Even the tough young dude who becomes gray haired one day. The wisdom of experience and heartbreak teaches compassion, which is passed on to younger men. Respecting Father Time and your natural cycle of life is psychological acceptance that allows for the potential of living our best life. Your mental health starts with understanding your body's messages and signals to you.

Let's take a timeout to consider some of the more obvious and not-so-obvious signs of male health and contemplate another side of the mind-body dynamic.

Psychological fact: Denial breeds confusion; acceptance breeds potential!

It is common knowledge in the medical field that women are more likely to seek out medical attention prior to a physical crisis than men. Dr. Mills so accurately stated in his quote at the beginning of this chapter that men (me included) tend to seek out medical treatment as a reaction (erectile dysfunction or body part falling off) rather than a preventive measure. When your knee isn't moving, penis is not working properly, or we are knocked out with the flu, it's amazing how we suddenly find time to make that doctor's appointment. The reasons vary; men avoid their health because they don't have time, money, or a good doctor. Before we go any further, I want to recommend an excellent book for practical, male-oriented medical practices: *A Field Guide to Men's Health*, by Dr. Mills, explores science and medical issues surrounding men's physical health. Dr. Mills addresses some common medical questions that men have and do not ask about regarding testosterone, diet, sexual functioning, prostate cancer, and many more. Science and all aspects of men's mental health are interwoven. You can't separate white and red blood cells and say they are independent of each other any more than you can separate your mental health from your physical health—it's impossible.

We focus on decoding your body's signals to you—positive, troubling, or whatever is happening in your outside or inside life. The catch is to be pro-active and recognize that something might be off in your life on more levels than just the physical. Your body is a complex system that interacts with all of you—it sounds obvious until he (your body) stops performing at its normal pace-level of excellence. Your emotions, mental processes, thoughts, eating, sleeping, and work life are all teammates on your field of life. These players literally and figuratively combine, creating your own mind-body mental health fitness level. Ultimately at some point in your life, this powerful connection within will grab your full attention. No one is exempt. Don't be scared if your health isn't perfect; things happen along the way in your life.

Medical truism: The term disease literally means the absence of ease within your body, that your body isn't functioning properly.

The study of the mind-body connection dates back to ancient Chinese medicine more than five thousand years ago. This idea of the mind-body relationship isn't new but a dynamic for men to embrace. Why the interest then and today? Eastern medicine and now Western medicine recognize that all the elements in your life impact each other. The term *disease* literally means that there is imbalance and uneasiness with your mind-body system. The disharmony creates all types of issues for men besides physical—relational, professional, family, financial, health, sexual, and personal. The list of variables is endless as is the impact on your day-to-day routine, choices, and future.

MEN'S FEAR AND AVOIDANCE OF MEDICINE: A COMMON SPOKEN AND UNSPOKEN ISSUE

I address some of the perplexing questions about men's medical health that most men dismiss as trivial and irrelevant in their day-to-day life until they are sick in bed. The terms such as "heartbreak" and "emotionally crushed" are now recognized as mental and physical health issues for men. Over the years, I have had several men experience the onset of cardiac arrest (heart attack) in my office while talking about an ex-wife, a heartbreaking experience, or a significant romantic loss. The sudden onset of physical symptoms come on in a serious, painful, frighting manner.

My male clients, ages twenty-eight, thirty-six, and forty-four, were all in seemingly good health then suddenly felt enormous chest pain pressure (like someone was sitting on their chest), tingling sensation in their arms, and shortness of breath. All three men wondered out loud if they were having a heart attack or a panic attack. Their physical symptoms began escalating—more chest pain and dizziness. The panic attack idea was dismissed by all three men, who had previously suffered them. Each of these men immediately sought emergency medical treatment; ironically, they had no hesitation seeking medical help in that moment.

Fortunately, getting immediate medical attention saved each of their lives, per their own admission in the following months. At the onset of their heart attacks, all three men were discussing their feelings of anger, hopelessness, and psychological loss when their bodies signaled trouble. It's interesting to note that each of the guys told me later that they had felt similar physical and emotional sensations days prior to their heart attacks and ignored them.

Question 1: Have You Noticed a Physical Sensation in Your Body while Talking about Emotionally Charged Issues?

Full disclosure: I am included among the majority of men who postpone their preventive medical care. Like the majority of the brotherhood, I didn't have time; my insurance deductible was high; I was building my psychological practice; and whatever excuses worked. I tore my vertebral artery at the base of my neck running and had a stroke that almost ended my life. I was completely paralyzed on the right side of my body within ten seconds. I knew I was dying (people know this during a near-death experience) and internally pleaded with my higher self to spare my life.

During the first forty-eight hours, I fortunately regained about 95 percent of my movement. I spent the following eight days in the intensive care unit, which felt like eight months. Needless to say, every doctor I met during my week in the hospital lectured me. They all told me how lucky I was not to be permanently paralyzed or dead (all movement fully came back to my body within a week). This medical crisis changed the course of my life; the psychological issues of avoidance, maintaining proper health, work-life balance, father-son issues, and a host of buried issues all resurfaced as I lay in the hospital.

After my brush with death, I had to ask myself what else was I running from. All that I knew when I left the hospital was that I never wanted to have a stroke—or anything like it—again. It took six months before I felt as if I was fully back in my body again.

Think about the three questions posed in this chapter. What is your first answer—not the proper response but the one in your gut? Make a mental note of your answer or write in the margin or at the end of this chapter. These questions can be helpful in reconnecting with lost or forgotten parts of your life. Your body is as important as your ability to think clearly and to function personally and professionally at your highest level.

Question 2: What Is Your Body Currently Saying to You?

Getting back to our mind-body connection is part of the masculine journey of developing balance and fulfillment, which all men address at some point in their lives. Women are typically more attuned to their bodies with monthly reminders about having babies someday. Men tend to rely on a crisis to address their health (both body and dental), as I am guilty of doing.

Years ago in California, smoking was allowed indoors, in restaurants, and basically anywhere else. Then legislators realized, per the medical community, that second-hand cigarette smoke was also a public health hazard, along with smoking. The concept of smoking and nonsmoking sections in restaurants, bars, and nightclubs was introduced. Within a short period of time, it became abundantly clear that smoke permeated any area regardless of ventilation. The conclusion: it is impossible to prevent cigarette smoke from filtering into other areas of a room. Soon, all public indoor smoking was banned in California. The take-away message of this obvious issue is that you cannot separate smoke from the nonsmoking areas—it simply does not work. Nor can we separate our emotional, psychological, and mental health from our physical health—it is simply not possible. Hence your mind-body connection is impossible to separate.

Your mental health and your physical health cannot be separated.

Chinese medicine is based on this fundamental truth: everything in a person's life is interconnected; it is a fluid operating system, interacting to create a harmonious balanced life. When there is disharmony in a person's system (i.e., unresolved personal issues, illness, money worries, dating, and endless life factors), this imbalance creates disease within the body over time. It is a scientific principle that all systems within an organism work together for the good of the whole. Gentlemen, we are not any different!

Operating like a robot isn't sustainable long term; you can't live your life in your head. Being a cerebral guy isn't bad, but it can't be your only option to function emotionally and relationally. Your feelings matter; the deliberate or unconscious avoidance of them eventually leads to catastrophe, such as the loss of relationships with your children, poor health, isolation, divorce, rage, contempt toward your family or partner, and an overall unhappy life. Over the years, countless men have sat in my office who were extremely wealthy (i.e., billionaires) and professionally powerful but emotionally and psychologically bankrupt.

Imbalance will always "break" our system of living to get us back to being balanced!

You can't work fourteen hours a day, drink only coffee or energy drinks, eat fast food, skip sleep, argue with the competition, and expect a good emotional outcome. Our lives are a composite of multiple factors, and these factors together produce a healthy life. Our bodies crave homeostasis: our natural state is health, balance, and smooth interactions. Western medicine acknowledges underlying psychological issues, unseen casualties of emotional upset, early life traumas, depression, and chronic anxiety and their collateral damage on the physical body.

> *Yo, I need some fucking help! Those six words changed my life!*
> —John Wald, NBA All Star discussing how he dealt with physical injuries that affected his mental health

John Wald is a great example of a man who is rich, gifted, famous, and not invincible. Experiencing a possible career-ending knee injury and the enormous struggles that come with physical recovery is dauting. Most of us think that we are the only ones who struggle with physical and emotional issues. Regardless of their situation in life, men are more similar to each other than they are dissimilar. John Wald is an example of our commonality, not exclusivity. No man is beyond his body's needs and wants.

Question 3: How Am I Creating Physical and Emotional Balance in My Life?

In sports, men readily accept that emotional loss impacts a team's performance in the next game or the next season. Why are we any different? We are not. Our physical well-being is directly impacted by our feelings, thoughts (critical or positive), choices, actions, life events, stress, losses, money worries, personal beliefs, and lifestyle. The point is that men of all ages have psychological feelings that connect to our physical well-being.

For instance, it is very difficult to get up Monday morning when your girlfriend ended your two-year relationship over the weekend via a text message. It is difficult to fall asleep even though you are physically exhausted, worrying about your rent payment due in three days, and currently unemployed.

These naturally occurring mind-body connections seem basic and obvious, yet they can cause profound health issues.

Men and change are not usually good friends until our nemesis, despair, shows up with a cancer diagnosis or a stroke (in my case). Despair is the driving force for men to become disciplined, motivated, and proactive about changing their lifestyle and mental health.

WHAT ARE PSYCHOSOMATIC ILLNESSES? AM I THE PROBLEM?

You have a powerful mind-body connection, hence the concept of psycho-somatic medicine. This field of medicine has been gaining popularity along with holistic medicine since the 1980s. The idea is that emotional experiences (good or bad) and their expression (the ability to describe and talk about them) play an invaluable role in a man's physical and psychological health. Likewise, suppression (conscious or unconscious) or avoidance of painful emotional topics (i.e., Roy avoids his rage about his father) or traumatic events past or present can be a major factor in a man's illnesses as much as a genic predisposition to it.

These correlations are now widely accepted by the scientific community along with medical researchers. Psychologists have long known that emotional avoidance buries the painful feeling within the body. Eventually the issue re-surfaces at some point, usually during a personal crisis. Psychosomatic ill-nesses can be described as a mental health crisis that is negatively impacting your physical health.

MIKE'S HEALTH ISSUES: MARIJUANA AND ANGER

Young men typically coast into their early or mid-twenties without many health problems or illness. For example, Mike, age twenty-five, believes that there is no psychological or physical connection between his angry outbursts, raging arguments with his family, heavy marijuana use, resentment toward his boss, and his chronic immunity issues.

In Mike's mind, he has "bad" DNA from his parents and his emotional vol-atility is a separate issue. Mike reports that he was full of energy prior to age eighteen with no health issues. He started smoking and vaping marijuana daily during his freshman year of college. Mike does not want to believe that his health issues could be impacted by his mental state of mind. Mike adamantly argues with me that his family issues and habitual drug use are independent of his current health challenges. I beg to differ with Mike. I reminded him that he has control and influence over his body and emotions. His response to that mind-body idea: "Doc, you are crazy. My issues aren't that bad; it's my awful parents who gave me bad genes." Mike is currently committed to his inner narrative that his parents are the problems in his life—not his heavy use of pot—contributing to his poor health.

Mike is committed to his position of blaming his parents and circumstances and unwilling to accept any responsibility. I mention to Mike that a classic side effect of heavy marijuana use is THC-induced rage, mood swings, and emotional instability. Mike canceled all future appointments with me.

DO I HAVE PSYCHOSOMATIC ISSUES?

The practice of medicine is an ongoing science with new discoveries each year. The medical model of science of the body to the exclusion of the whole person is no longer the prevailing practice in Western medicine. Doctors now consider a person's psychosocial and psychological factors as part of their overall health, treatment, history, and care. Consider the emotional, psychological, and personal components of the life events and issues listed below in relation to your long-term health. Some common psychological and psychosocial medical health issues that can impact your life include:

- Being laid off or terminated at work; unemployment—feeling despair, alone, dismissed, rejected
- Divorce process, child custody issues, coparenting, or loss of a meaningful relationship—feeling like "damaged goods"
- Marriage, blended family challenges, in-laws—hope, anxiety, changing life plans, relocation stress
- College graduation—sense of achievement, fear of the future, anxiety about a life plan or finding a job/career?
- Moving, either locally or across the country; roommate problems—avoiding change, feeling relieved
- Children leaving or returning from school—sadness, excitement
- Aging parents; living with your parents—fear of loss/death, acceptance
- Suffering a physical injury or chronic illness—depression, doom, dread of the unknown
- Death of a partner, close childhood friend, emotional support animal—grief, loss, hopelessness
- No close friends at work or in your private life—feelings of hopelessness, regret, despair (suicidal thoughts)
- Chronic worry/stress about money, career, and relationships—nothing feels secure or safe, mood swings due to despair
- Bankruptcy, foreclosure, or loss of retirement fund—feeling socially isolated, shame, regret about prior choices
- Having a baby—natural, adopted, or via surrogacy—feeling excitement, overwhelmed, sleep deprived, lacking a support network

These are some of the typical events and situations and related emotions that can be triggered in your everyday life. Change and disruption of your emotional (how you feel) and mental (how you think) balance is normal and not unique to you—it is common but rarely discussed among men. Again, the old masculine model that a strong man can express only anger and calmness in the face of fear isn't helpful or useful. Uncovering these unspoken beliefs within you about your own personal "gag order" is healing and life changing.

Question 4—What Situation, Event, or Relationship Could Be Impacting My Health Currently?

In the practice of psychology, it isn't the events that are a mental health concern. Rather, how we react to these events is a big determinate of our mental and physical well-being. Men typically live in their heads—emotionally disconnected from their life events.

For instance, when anxious or stressed about money, your body has a physical reaction to it. Anxiety, like all emotional reactions, has a physical component to which your brain and body respond. For example, you might suddenly feel your heart racing or experience stomach/indigestion issues when you attempt to manage your money concerns, dating expectations, friend circle, or professional colleagues. A hot topic for men is family relationships past and present. These critical emotional bonds are anything but neutral or avoidable for men.

Question 5—Do I Accept the Fact That I Had or Am Having Emotionally and Mentally Challenging Events in My Life?

The list of events mentioned are only some of the common stressors men face and generally dismiss as trivial. The point isn't to throw a pity party but rather to clearly understand how you manage the uncomfortable things in your life. The problem with emotional denial, avoidance, and suppression of your feelings past or present is that they will break down your body. Severe mind-body traumatic situations can lead to serious health issues and, in some cases, death.

Our bodies and emotions never sleep—they are always on.

Our bodies aren't sleeping when we are—resting and healing, yes, but not sleeping. Our bodies are on the clock from the moment we joined this life and until the day we depart it. Our emotions, thoughts, and feelings are energies that our psychological and physical bodies manage 24/7—prenatally to the present moment. The control center of your body is your brain, and the corporate headquarters is your frontal lobe (forehead area), which is where your best life is lived, understood, and managed. Our brain reacts to our emotions with a variety of chemicals and physical movements. The superpower of your fight-or-flight adrenaline pump is discussed here and throughout the book. Many psychosomatic illnesses are based in the chronic fight/flight responses to your day-to-day life. *Your quality of living matters more than the quantity of living.* Think about that.

Although we know that dinosaurs are no longer chasing us, our internal response to a call from our boss can elicit the same biochemical reactions in our body—fear for our life (lose our job and our life is over). Long-term exposure to adrenaline (a stress hormone) breaks down and dysregulates the normal physiological functioning of our bodies—imbalance again. This pattern of overreacting to all concerns, whether significant or minor, can trigger binge eating, heavy alcohol drinking, recreational drug use, and sexual impulsivity.

ROADBLOCKS TO YOUR HEALTH—YOU

We met Roy at the beginning of this chapter. Per his own self-analysis, Roy is a steroid-using, professionally driven, money motivated bodybuilder who hates authority, has not spoken to his father in more than three years, and, at times, is verbally aggressive toward his girlfriend. Roy woke up one morning with severe pain in his lower back area. The pain throbbed and burned. Roy went to the emergency room knowing something was terribly wrong with his body. He could barely walk.

After more than five hours in the ER, the doctor advised Roy that he had a severe liver infection, enlarged prostate, dangerously high blood pressure, and an irregular heartbeat. He asked Roy if he was using any type of steroid or growth hormones. Roy explained that he had been injecting himself twice a week with a steroid that he bought from his college buddy who works out at his gym.

Upon hearing of Roy's long-term use of steroids (more than five months), the doctor immediately hospitalized him for the next nine days. During that time, Roy had several MRIs to check for any tumors or blood clots in his body. Several blood clots were found in his legs.

Roy and I spoke on the phone while he was in the hospital, and I asked him who he had unfinished business with. Roy promised me that he would call his father after we hung up and break the icy silence between them. Roy was scared that he might die and felt powerless to keep his body from shutting down.

Roy called his father. They spoke for a few minutes, and his father, who lives on the East Coast, said he was flying to Los Angeles immediately to see him. Roy's dad, Mark, arrived later that day, and they cried and hugged each other. Both men regretted allowing their differences to interfere with their relationship. This crisis got Roy to address his "rage" and resentment toward his father since childhood.

Roy admitted he knew that his steroid use, poor choices, and aggressive behaviors stemmed from his unresolved relationship with his father. Roy needed this medical crisis, which almost killed him, to force him to face his emotional past, which was hindering him from living his life. Roy was fortunate to survive his physical and emotional neglect. The power of our "rage" can be fatal if left unchecked; it caused Roy's hospitalization. Once our lives are abruptly stopped by our bodies' refusal to cooperate with our "wrong" choices, we find the courage to address what seemed impossible the day before.

Taking action is critical for any significant change in life—what's your next move?

Any degree of change requires us to make emotional and mental commitments to our overall quality of life, mental health, and balanced masculinity. I discuss with my clients the following questions and topics as a beginning point for creating a healthier mind-body connection:

- Your physical health is not in a vacuum. All the facets of your life are an ongoing interaction of variables. What emotions, thoughts, people, and circumstances in your past and present do you dismiss?
- What is your foundational "glue" that guides your life?
- What influence does your body have in your daily life?
- Your physical health can be an indicator of other issues in your life requiring your attention. What physical symptoms or physical aches and pains do you experience?
- Do you believe that your mental health spills into your physical health?
- There are no dividing lines among your body, mind, and emotions. All three parts of you interact 24/7 all the days of your life.
- Do you allow yourself to rest, pause, and stop emotionally moving during your workweek?

- What can you do to create more balance between your work life and time spent with your family, friends, and alone?
- Bodybuilding, running, skiing, rock climbing, and walking involves movement. What things do you do to connect with your body?
- Men account for the highest rate of preventable deaths according to the National Institute of Health. What behaviors, actions, or choices do you make that are dangerous?

CHAPTER TWO

THE NARCISSISTIC MASCULINE TYPE

You Are More Than Your Body, Your Looks,
and Your Athleticism

Unexpressed emotions will never die. They are buried alive and will come forth later in uglier ways.—Dr. S. Freud, father of psychotherapy

Males represent 25% of individuals with anorexia nervosa, and they are at a higher risk of dying in part because they are often diagnosed later since many people assume males don't have eating disorders. —J. M. Mond, D. Mitchison, and P. Hay, *International Journal of Eating Disorders* (2014)

MALE NARCISSISM AND TOXIC MASCULINITY—A CLOSE FRIENDSHIP

No one would argue that the term "narcissist" is unusual for a certain type of teenage boy, dude, or adult man. We all know these guys, or maybe our partner, friends, or ex-lovers have told us that we are that guy. If men are honest, no one wants to be *that* guy. That particular guy ultimately lives on an island all by himself; it's a sad story but nonetheless a hot topic socially, corporately, legally, and personally. The male masculinity crisis—male role confusion—is in large part due to the toxic nature of this all-too-common male-dominated me-first psychological dynamic. Fueling the confusion is Peter Pan syndrome, which is part and parcel to the masculine crisis of narcissism. A large percentage of the married women seeking marriage counseling come to my office with a unifying complaint of being "fed up," exhausted from being their husbands' or boyfriends' surrogate mothers. These woman—from their late twenties to their seventies—all say the same thing: "When is he going to get it and grow up?"

Women want a man, not an overgrown teenager who is forty-two and wants her financial support until he figures out his life. You may ask—as I did—why did these women allow their partner to "coast" in the first place. Again, a common theme among these kind, faithful, and resentful women emerged; they believed that he would grow up, get his act together, and become the man they always believed he could be.

Unfortunately, their partners haven't launched and, in most cases, became less helpful with the kids and their life together, and the women lost respect for their partners. In chapters 11 and 12, I discuss how to recover your relationship when your partner has lost respect for you—it's possible to repair.

This type of man is often referred to as a "man-child" because of his immaturity and lack of psychological growth. There is never-ending unspoken emotional neediness for the approval and nurturing of the wife/partner/significant other. These men, regardless of sexual orientation, haven't developed the psychological ability to reciprocate the nurturing or to think of others before themselves. They are consumed with their issues, needs, and unfair treatment by the world. During the relationship, the partner becomes an object of disdain by the narcissistic male for not "fixing" his issues. It is paradoxical and completely irrational that the wife, girlfriend, or romantic partner becomes the object of disdain by the narcissistic man.

Let's keep this discussion from becoming too dry and clinical: it's important to know that narcissistic men have not developmentally separated from their mothers. They crave her approval well past childhood and still need constant emotional nurturing and her permission to make his own life decisions. This might sound a little wild, but it is one of the primary driving forces behind the maladaptive masculine narcissistic model.

The emotional maturity level for those with any form of addiction, unresolved traumas, and untreated narcissism is age fifteen.

The arrested development—emotional immaturity—of a narcissistic man is that of a fifteen-year-old boy. Psychology also considers age fifteen the emotional age of people with any addictive behaviors—drinking, gambling, sexual, smoking, and so forth. Healthy male psychological growth progresses through this stage of life and learns to embrace empathy, compassion, purpose, and passion for the importance of life—the four primary features of the new masculinity. Men with narcissistic tendencies are driven by the need to be important or to know important people, to behave as if they are invincible physically (i.e., using heroin, behaving recklessly) with no regard for the consequences of their choices or actions. Consequences don't apply to the self-absorbed man. This type of man believes that the rules of life or the legal system, do *not* apply to them. They are bigger than life and everyone should know it. This sounds obnoxious, and it is the tragic plight of these lost boys in men's bodies. These guys are walking around telling the world to follow them off the cliff of ignorance and despair.

The stories of Wall Street tycoons who steal billions of dollars from retirement accounts, misusing trusted funds, are prime examples of narcissistic boys in men's bodies, driving million-dollar cars to the gym. Let's first formally define narcissism for our purposes and how it relates to men's masculine development. It's important to note that narcissism expresses itself differently in women and the distinction here is solely for purposes of clarifying the male identity crisis (see chapter 9). Also, the reference to a female partner is for literary purposes and does not exclude any type of romantic bond between two men. Relationships, love, immaturity, narcissism, mental health, eating disorders, self-acceptance, and masculinity aren't selective or exclusive in how they function in a man's life or relationship with his significant other. The dynamics are universal; it is only the circumstances that are as varied as the people involved.

Working definition of male narcissism: Male narcissism exhibits itself with an exaggerated sense of importance, grandiose ideas about themselves that simultaneously mask their low self-esteem; self-centered thinking that lacks empathy; a view of things in their world as important only if those things directly relate to them; the distorted perspective of life that everything is about them even when it is not; a chronic need or craving to be seen and noticed. Male narcissists dominate conversations and make every story event about them; need to be admired and seek constant emotional reassurance; are prone to fits of rage when their needs are not met; are inclined toward physical violence and domestic violence toward family and partner; view people as objects; are verbally and emotionally abusive and demeaning to others, especially intimate partners, close friends, and family members; want and have the emotional need to dominate, always to be in a position of power regardless of the consequences to others; value status, popular brands, looking perfect, and being admired by others; are vain about body image, weight, and aging. The value of their appearance far exceeds the value of inner personal meaning, mental health, and inner personal challenges. Male narcissists are only as good as they look, the cars they drive, the money they make, the house they own, and whatever premium they value.

The narcissist masculinity crisis does not discriminate based on sexual orientation, race, education, wealth, privilege, or family background. It is a universal challenge for all men.

This a practical description (see the bibliography for more detailed information about the psychology of narcissism) of these types of men, who range anywhere from age sixteen to one hundred years old, which highlights the lifelong struggles of their masculine character flaws. The chronic need to compensate for any feelings of inadequacy is a driving force that these men inherently battle every day of their life. (Yes, this man can be healed of his self-absorbed masculine paradigm; see chapters 13, 14, and 15.) Men trapped in this self-defeating masculine maze use any circumstance or opportunity to advance their cause and public image.

The lack of concern for others in the workplace, for instance, is dismissed as business only—absent of concern or empathy for the individual. Cutthroat behavior is not personal; it is about money or power. The irony of life is that everything is personal, regardless of the setting or circumstances—your life is a matrix of personal relationships! Relationships matter and they can never be dismissed or trivialized as unimportant. I discuss the balance between wealth, business, profitability, and being a gracious colleague later.

Narcissistic masculinity is a continual battle to be seen as physically perfect with no emotional problems past or present!

The appearance-driven man comes in many shapes, sizes, and severities. Everything in life is based on degrees of severity—80 percent gray and 10 percent black and 10 percent white at the extremes. The self-reporting questionnaire below is designed to ask the difficult questions about your personality blind spots (we all have them), self-loathing and self-acceptance, psychological vulnerability, punitive behaviors, and the people in your life. This type of male personality has to be surrounded by passive and accepting men. These men supportive of the narcissist oftentimes struggle with their own imposter syndrome—inadequacy and not feeling "good enough"—and fall prey to domineering bigger-than-life friends and colleagues with overpowering personalities. Narcissistic men are driven by the need to appear perfect inside and outside. These self-centered, seemingly masculine men surround themselves with men who suffer from self-doubt, fear of rejection, and a history of being bullied. The narcissistic man is chronically needy and finds passive male friends and lovers

THE NARCISSISTIC MASCULINE TYPE **21**

who placate his psychological issues. The passive men are also seeking validation, which was withheld from them in their childhood. The narcissistic friendship is based on superficiality and looking cool, accomplished, or whatever measurement this group of men use.

TAKE-HOME TEST OF HONESTY—
A PERSONAL LOOK IN THE MIRROR

Answer the following questions with a "yes" or "no." There are no wrong answers to your personal inventory of your life today. These questions are strictly for you to begin to see your psychological and relational blind spots. The defensive wall of masculine pain protected you when you were younger to keep you "safe." Now, as an adult man, this barbwire covering a brick wall of fear is no longer functional and creates more problems in your life than it solves. The outdated mode of psychological functioning has to be updated from the inside if any significant change is going to happen. The narcissistic wall (we all have walls) might be covered up with years and years of denial, unresolved disappointment, abuse, or traumatic events in your past. Your personal walls are not trivial; they are a vital part of who you are and how you operate in your life today and every day, for that matter.

The false "bravado" is a self-serving element that keeps men (you and me) from ever feeling vulnerable or truly honest with ourselves and others—again, this is inclusive of all men regardless of age, culture, life experience, income potential, or career. The problem with this very common masculine wall of unresolved psychological issues is that it keeps you isolated and prevents you from healing and resolving the seemingly unresolvable mental health challenges (nothing is unresolvable) in your past and present day.

Narcissistic men are lonely and desperately hoping someone can help them find their way out of their maze of pain and inadequacy—their greatest fear and greatest wish! Keep reading because we have to first recognize this wall in its many forms in order to understand it and rebuild your life from within. The masculine journey takes us into our dark cave where our deepest secrets, fears, traumas, treasures, dreams, and hopes are hidden. The phrase "don't get dark" comes from this idea of our deepest truths are within us and we have to go into our inner cave.

1. Do you hide your true feelings and disappointments from your inner circle of friends? *Yes or no.*
2. Is it difficult for you to apologize when you know you are wrong or when you hurt someone's feelings? *Yes or no.*

3. Do you keep all your relationships at arm's length? *Yes or no.*

4. Do you privately wish ill to those who have hurt or disappointed you in the past and present—for example, in your career, personal life, ex-lovers? *Yes or no.*

5. Are you rude and demeaning to customer service people, restaurant workers, or anyone you deem as "less than"? *Yes or no.*

6. Do you tell people about your successes only—never about your struggles, self-doubts, or fears? *Yes or no.*

7. You view humility as a psychological weakness, not a character strength? *Yes or no.*

8. Would your coworkers describe you as "ruthless," a monster, or someone who is dangerous to upset? *Yes or no.*

9. Does your family and close friends avoid telling you the truth about yourself to prevent your explosive verbal or physical reaction? *Yes or no.*

10. Do you believe that men with mental health issues are just seeking attention or excuses for not working harder? *Yes or no.*

11. Have you ever been told by your romantic partner that you are "self-centered" and only care about yourself? *Yes or no.*

12. Do you surround yourself with yes-men in your relationships? *Yes or no.*

13. Do you tend to blame others for your mistakes? *Yes or no.*

14. Do you have a relationship history of being unfaithful to your partner, cheating, womanizing, or seducing others? *Yes or no.*

15. Does your partner accuse you of not taking responsibility for your self-centered actions and self-motivated decisions in the relationship? *Yes or no.*

16. Do you drink and black out or use cocaine and related drugs regardless of their health consequences or impact on your relationships? *Yes or no.*

17. Do you hold grudges or aggressively retaliate against perceived enemies when you can? *Yes or no.*

18. Do you habitually lie to embellish your status and reputation and to avoid responsibility? *Yes or no.*

19. Have you been accused of having explosive mood swings or verbally aggressive raging episodes? *Yes or no.*

20. Do you feel cheated by the system, your company, your parents, your lover, and life in general? *Yes or no.*

These questions are specifically designed to help you to consider your personality, relationships, and ability to be transparent. Your close circle of friends might be worth taking a look at; do you control them or ignore their needs or suggestions?

What is one question from the list above that you found irritating or helpful and why? Many times, the things that bother us the most in others are the very issues that we don't see or want to see in ourselves. Why are we critical of these qualities in others? The short answer is that we see the unhealed narcissistic parts of ourselves in that other guy—and he sucks. Take moment. Think about who you thoroughly dislike or even despise. Now, focus on what bugs you about this guy. Chances are *his* arrogance or personality issue is something about you or in you that isn't resolved.

I know this question and the other twenty questions asked are blunt, harsh, honest, and necessary. It's normal to reject or ignore the things we don't want to address in our past and present-day struggles. Remember, you would not be reading this book if you were not interested in knocking down the outdated walls of pain in your life! Finally, denial and avoidance are some of the strongest emotional responses inside of you when you are vulnerable and moving toward changing your psychological perspective, which is something to think about.

> *I am not what happened to me, I am what I chose to become.*
> —Dr. Carl Jung

The psychological principle I discuss and present throughout this book is referred to as Jungian psychology—founded by Dr. Carl Jung (1875–1961). It is based on the premise that we project our unconscious traumas and unresolved issues onto others who—consciously or unconsciously—have the same wounds and untreated shame/psychological issues that we do. It's the strong, visceral disdain that we have for someone else that is a signal that we struggle with a similar personality flaw or emotional issue. Carl Jung is the founder and pioneer of this deep-healing psychoanalytic emotional work.

A CAUTIONARY TALE—UNTREATED MALE NARCISSISM

Dean, age twenty-seven and single, grew up in the South and came to California after the COVID-19 shutdown during the spring of 2021 to pursue a career in the entertainment business. Prior to coming to Los Angeles, Dean dropped out of college in his third year and moved to Aspen, Colorado, and became a ski instructor. He fell (his words) into a fast crowd of partiers who recreationally used cocaine, heroin, Valium, and OxyContin (a muscle relaxer)—all highly addictive and dangerous drugs. Dean left Aspen for Los Angeles and began taking acting classes. He wanted to get away from the drug culture and his friends in Colorado. To support himself, Dean became a professional poker player. Dean entered several poker tournaments and shortly thereafter switched to using his smartphone for his day-to-day gambling. The poker tournaments were long and tiring for Dean; he wanted something faster. He started betting on any and all sports, ranging from professional and college football to high school sports. Dean, within six months, had an online gambling debt of more than $10,000 and owed several bookies another $30,000.

Dean kept gambling, believing he could win it all back. He had what he calls his "special powers" to win and knew when to bet. The adrenaline rush of winning was better than drugs or sex according to Dean. Additionally, he became obsessed with body art and had both arms, his back, and his legs completely covered in tattoos.

Recently, some employees of his bookie confronted Dean.

The confrontation was physical and they threatened his life if he didn't begin to pay back his losses. Dean called his parents, who bailed him out of this crisis and paid off his entire gambling debt to all parties involved. Dean was "pissed off" that his bookie forced him to pay back his losses sooner than he wanted—but he didn't mention his parent's generosity.

Men who are able to share their struggles with male friends find the emotional support healing and positive for their mental health.

Recently, Dean began experiencing erectile disfunction, and his girlfriend broke up with him several times (dramatic relationship), accusing him of having sex with other women. Dean was not cheating on her and had been experiencing serious physical side effects (i.e., abdominal pain, blood in urine, body aches) due to his prolific drug use since age twenty. His medical doctor referred Dean to me to address his impulsivity, sexual issues, steroid use, eating disorder, and sense of invincibility. Dean is currently sober and no longer gambling.

TEAM SPORTS AND MALE BONDING— WHY IT MATTERS FOR YOUR MENTAL HEALTH

The topic of men and sports could be its own building at the Library of Congress for endless reasons. The ability to share the experience of your team psychologically, emotionally, and physically beating your archrival is a unifying experience. Alumni of the same college emotionally share their common dislike for their crosstown rival with no regard for social standing or different friend groups. Professional sports bring together men from all walks of life to experience several hours of unity. Going to a stadium, a sports bar, or a friend's house wearing their favorite jersey allows men to step away from their day-to-day life and be with other men. Sports unite men with a common purpose, reason, and goal: winning. The competition is third person, not a direct ego-versus-ego standoff between members of the same fan base. Men are pack animals, and we love to be part of a team.

Sports create a level playing field for all men, including the narcissistic guy, who can experience a sense of belonging on (or rooting for) his team. Traditional settings such as work, running, golfing, and coaching your child's team lend themselves to individual competition and comparisons: who is better?

For example, many years ago while coaching Little League baseball for my son's team, two fathers—both exceedingly wealthy, smart, and narcissistic—got into a physical altercation while discussing the postgame with me. I told my son to get into the car so he would not witness the fight, a classic male meltdown. I got between the two men and walked one of them away, explaining that the disagreement didn't matter. This coach, a former Major League All Star baseball player, stopped and screamed at me, "It fucking matters! Mike [the other coach] can't push me around or think he knows more than I do about baseball!" I continued to walk the coach out of the parking lot, attempting to explain that we are all on the same team with the same goals for our sons. Neither coach at that moment was remotely receptive to talking and avoiding a fistfight. It should be noted that each of these men were in their late forties.

Both coaches later told me they struggle with depression. Some of the common but misunderstood signs of a mood disorder such as depression presents in men as rage, irritability, and aggressiveness. As a result of their altercation, both men were banned from going to or participating in any Little League baseball games for five years.

Male depression is often disguised as anger, irritability, physical violence, and verbal aggressiveness.

Sports remove that invisible layer of insecurity and create an immediate psychological bond between strangers that otherwise is difficult for men to achieve or experience. The thrill of watching your favorite team or player winning or losing with a group of likeminded men is a wonderful supportive group dynamic for men. Throughout human history, men are pack animals that do well connected to a pack, group, or common cause. One of the amazing powers of Alcoholic Anonymous (AA) is the universal acceptance of anyone, regardless of life situation—men thrive with group support. Men who are connected to a group of men via sports, biking, running, a hobby, a charity,

Men thrive when they have their own tribe of likeminded men. Women know this about the value of the sisterhood.

or a spiritual organization report a higher level of happiness, supportive friends, sense of fulfillment, and a better quality of relationships.

Since the beginning of time, men have needed a community. Women recognize this fact and are great at creating their own network of support and sisterhood with loving girlfriends. Women do book clubs together, walking groups, and mommy-and-me groups for the collective support of other females. Men need the same type of psychological connection. The sense of belonging to something bigger than yourself is a transformational experience for a man's mental health and self-worth. Oftentimes, in marriage or any type of long-term romantic union, men begin to lean exclusively on their wife/partner for all of their social, emotional, and friendship needs. This creates an out-of-balance psychological issue for men. The need for men to have their own tribe of likeminded men has given rise to men's groups, weekend retreats, workshops strictly designed to help guys of all ages create new emotional bonds later in life.

Sole dependency on our wives or partners for all of our personal needs is a formula for disaster. It is one of the major stumbling blocks that men fall into—no one person can meet all our needs! Our partners resent this unspoken pressure to be "everything," which only breeds resentment in both parties.

Your romantic partner can't be your sole emotional support. No one relationship can meet all your needs.

The importance for men to have a close confidant, supportive buddy, or childhood friend is something that we are going to continually discuss, because it is a major element for the new masculinity and men's mental health. Same-sex relationships are different than opposite-sex relationships—obviously. But this is not as apparent to men as one would think. This is why sports (noncompetitive in nature) and being part of a community is critical for men's mental health and an antidote against male depression and male suicide. The bottom line is that men cannot exist or thrive without each other.

TEAM SPORTS, ATHLETICS, GANGS, AND NARCISSISM— A RELATIONSHIP OF MALE CONFUSION

The purpose of our discussion is to explore the psychological impact that a few reckless men and boys perpetuate on the greater whole of society. Our discussion is much larger in scope than politics, race, and the lack of institutional accountability often evaded by male leadership. Our focus is on the grassroots-level lack of accountability among men.

The "herd" mentality of conformity to team rules, fraternities, businesses, and rituals is fast becoming a hornet's nest of problems, which isn't unwarranted. It's the emotional, mental, physical, and psychological abuse perpetuated in the name of team unity that is no longer kept secret by the brotherhood. These male-driven initiation/hazing traditions are now being called into question regarding their purpose and intention of their goals.

Men who cross the line of initiation into the areas of humiliation, sexual abuse of others, or any type of "hazing" are now being exposed. This outdated male model of creating unity through abuse is problematic for the majority of younger men, who don't see the purpose or reason for it. Younger men (under thirty-five years old) want to enjoy the team camaraderie, spirit of unity, and belonging to a group without the old-school mentality and physical abuse. The goodwill and emotional support among men is never the problem; it's the old traditions employed without question or reason. Men closely relating through a shared activity is empowering for men and their personal psychological development. Men who isolate, who are loners, or who fear being bullied are at the greatest risk for mental health issues.

The new masculinity of embracing the "complete man" doesn't include demeaning others in order to belong to the group. There is no benefit, despite the old-school argument of passing along tradition. The dysfunctional male mentality of secrecy in sports (i.e., ownership, coaching, staffing, and officiating) teams and clubs; college sports, both male and female; and teen sports organizations have been the subject of ongoing criminal investigations. Fraternities, hazing, and belonging to a team is as much a part of our culture as celebrating someone's birthday or successes. Football teams starting at the peewee level (ages nine through eleven years old) have a system of creating unity for these boys. The psychological motivation of "hazing" by teenage boys, college men, and professional athletics is alarming. We aren't going to get lost in this all-important topic of men, violence against women and others, and the need to be part of a winning team. The "old masculine" model of narcissism, control, power, and abuse perpetuate this problematic framework, which is no longer acceptable by men. It is absolutely possible to create a supportive climate mentally, physically, and emotionally without violating everyone along the way to the championship. I

A wise man once said, "Show me your friends and I will show you your future!"

don't mean to sound extreme; if we are talking about men, then we are also talking about sports. The problems of men and sports are only symptoms of the underlying need for healthy masculinity.

Lifetime of Benefits for Men Having Male Friends

Numerous research studies all point to the intrinsic value of male relationships for men and their myriad benefits, including:

- Friendships among men also improved the quality of their relationships with their wife/partner—they were emotionally secure and available to connect with her. Two-thirds of all marriages end because the wife reports her husband was emotionally unavailable to her; this is a consistent pattern in my clinical practice during thirty years of couples therapy. Women want their men to be emotionally capable of connecting, understanding, and being supportive.
- Men have a special bond with other men that their relationships with their wife, female friends, or romantic partner can't replace. Men need men.
- Men with male friends (not the quantity but the in-depth quality) are less likely to become socially, personally, or psychologically isolated. Prolonged isolation can lead to stress-related illness, depression, addiction, suicide, divorce, and violence. Isolation is deadly for men.
- Men can offer suggestions and support to their friends to help increase their personal mental health resiliency during times of distress or crisis (e.g., loss of a job).
- Male friends, over a man's lifetime, improve their overall health and lessen the likelihood of Alzheimer's disease, obesity, diabetes, high blood pressure, heart disease, neurodegenerative diseases, and cancer. Relationships impact every area of a man's life: relationships matter.
- Having male friends leads to greater success in a man's personal and professional life; a positive attitude breeds success. Men who have a close male confidant do not feel alone or isolated and have the courage to confront issues that are normalized.

NARCISSISTIC SUMMARY AND IDEAS FOR BUILDING YOUR FUTURE

The new masculinity starts with embracing our psychological-behavioral blind spots. The need to see how we impact others for good or not so good are the beginning steps for healing our early childhood wounds and traumas. Dismantling the emotional wall of protection of our young self starts with the process of cognitively considering the opportunity of accepting loving gestures, acceptance, and understanding.

These three qualities are the unspoken universal needs of all men. The same guy who helped you with a flat tire in the rain could also be the same guy who steals your wallet or wife. All men crave the foundational core experience of "feeling okay." The healing process of a narcissistic man starts with exploring his past: feeling unloved, misunderstood, and rejected as a boy. These three core needs of love, understanding, and acceptance were not present, available, or part of a wounded man's childhood to the degree that he needed. We are going to deep dive into healing our past traumas, abuses, failures, and unspeakable secrets in the following chapters. But we have to identify the issues, pain, and trauma before we can heal and move forward—sorry, there are no shortcuts to balanced mental health and balanced masculinity.

"What are you holding on to?" and the questions that follow are designed to help you to see what is covered up or avoided because you might be too scared to ask about. Our painful narcissistic behaviors are a flashing red warning

> *Sage wisdom: You can't let go of what you don't know you are holding on to.*

light signaling our need to be understood, accepted, and loved. Men have an odd way of circumventing this process of healing with layers and layers of outrageous actions; 99.999 percent of all mass shootings are done by men.

These questions are for you to start cutting away the ivy-covered doorway to your mental health's freedom, personal empowerment, and fulfillment.

- What is one thing that you would like your male friends to understand about you?
- What is something about yourself that you have difficulty accepting?
- How do you show someone that you love them (including your partner)?
- Name a close friend from your childhood, teenage years, or adulthood whom you trust or trusted?
- With whom in your past or present do you have tension or unresolved issues?
- Who is a classic self-centered man in your life, past or present, who bothers you?
- What parts of his life bother you or remind you of things you don't like?

- What behaviors, attitudes, or success do the two of you share in common (tough question but be honest—there are some)?
- How does/did it feel to have a close friend or a few male friends with whom you share(d) your life?

FINALLY, DEAN'S PERSONAL CRISIS

Dean began coming to therapy as a condition for his parents paying off his gambling debt. After discussing his reckless behaviors, dangerous drug use, and risky betting, it became apparent that Dean didn't like himself. You can't run away from yourself forever. This might sound basic, but it is a profound insight. The self-loathing behaviors, narcissistic need to be the center of attention, and excessive tattoos all over his body were attempts to cover up his body dysmorphia. Dean always thought he was ugly. As a young boy Dean began to realize that at age five or six, he felt inferior to others, and this issue was never resolved.

Dean began to accept himself as he is, not as what he perceived as "cool," powerful, or rich. He no longer bases his self-worth on the car he drives, the home he lives in, or how much money he makes. These variables for Dean were a driving force for as long as he can remember. His sexual issues (performance) with his girlfriend dissipated. Dean slowly became more comfortable in his own skin and mindful that he doesn't need to be perfect inside and out. The relief of not trying to be "perfect" to the outside world was transformational for Dean. This lack of constantly comparing himself to others allowed him to be more compassionate and understanding of himself and others.

CHAPTER THREE

SEX, INTIMACY, SEXUAL PREFERENCE, AND MASCULINITY DEFINED

Gay, Straight, Bi, and You

The moment you accept yourself, you become beautiful.—Osho

Happiness can exist only with acceptance.—George Orwell

Male Body Fact 1: Men who have sex at least twice a week can reduce their risk of heart disease by almost half according to a 2010 study.

Male Body Fact 2: Men can boost their sex drive—it is possible. Some of the more common ways to increase your libido: diet, more sleep, emotional connection with your partner, limiting alcohol and drug use, reducing stress outside the bedroom, exercise, knowing your sex drive cycle, and acceptance of your sexual desires.

Male Body Fact 3: Despite what the adult film industry implies, only 15 percent of men have a penis longer than seven inches. Only 3 percent have a penis more than eight inches long. Your penis is not a measurement of masculinity, or your sexuality, or your ability to be sexual. Your sexuality is your choice, practice, and understanding.

Male Body Fact 4: Sex is considered one of the least-discussed stress busters for men (and women). It lowers your blood pressure, and the chemical release of an orgasm has a calming effect on your body, mind, and emotional perspective.

Male Body Fact 5: Hugging increases levels of the "love hormone," oxytocin. A hug lasting twenty seconds reduces the effects of stress and blood pressure. Additionally, human touch helps protect against illness, ease depression, and reduce pain. Hugging is invaluable for men, not just women. Men need the "human touch."

These fun facts about men's sexual behaviors, penis size, physical reactions, and chemical responses have nothing to do with sexual orientation or sexual preference—zero! Let's do a quick true-false test to establish our talking points and foundation for this all-important discussion of men, sex, sexual identity, sexual habits, body image, emotional intimacy, pornography, testosterone, and masculinity. These topics are all part and parcel to how men view and carry themselves every day at work, relating to friends, interacting with family, and navigating body image and romantic relationships. We are influenced by these variables and many more, which create and form the fabric of our sexuality, which is the expression of our masculine identity—it's all connected together.

For the purposes of our discussion, we focus on sexual preference, heterosexuality, homosexuality, and bisexuality, not sex changes or transgender and related topics. Although these topics are important and warrant their own examination, they are beyond the scope of our current discussion. Men secretly tune out emotionally during any discussion about sex that is outside their comfort zone, experience, or fund of knowledge. We focus on the more traditional sexual concerns for men here. The psychological discussions of medical and nonmedical sex changes are valuable and are beyond our scope in this book. This is without judgment, prejudice, or negative opinion.

It's socially assumed that if you are a man, then your sexuality is fully understood, developed, and complete. This statement couldn't be further from the truth. These types of generalized masculine themes cause more harm than good for men of all ages. We explore some of the foundational issues surrounding men and sex.

Our goal is to attempt to normalize the discussion and issues surrounding sex that goes beyond experiencing a life-changing orgasm. The social belief that men are basically sexually starved animals is a highly problematic perspective. This negative attitude about men and sex is inaccurate. Women and men both crave emotional connection and acceptance. The ingrained social beliefs about barbaric men and sex aren't useful or remotely helpful in creating a deeper understanding of masculinity and the sexuality component. The mental health mind-body issues, such as the psychological process of personal maturity and orientation (i.e., boys becoming men), is a valuable source of comfort and understanding for young men, single men, married men, gay men, bisexual men, and elderly men—no one is exempt. These foundational elements of sexual awareness are important for men to acknowledge regardless of their orientation or basis. Our discussion is inclusive; we simply focus on these particular areas of a man's sexual identity related to their masculinity.

SEXUALITY TRUE-FALSE QUESTIONS
FOR MEN AND ABOUT MEN

Please answer with your first thought and impression. Answer every question; there are *no* "I don't know" responses. Be honest with yourself for the purposes of furthering your sexual self-awareness—be courageous and say what you have maybe always thought but never articulated.

1. Sexual identity is a fixed issue, a permanent character quality and behavior for a man's entire life. *True or false?*
2. Sexual performance is different than sexual desire. *True or false?*
3. Women enjoy sex less than men. *True or false?*
4. Homosexuality is a mental disorder created by an overbearing maternal figure or absent father figure in a young boy's life. *True or false?*
5. Low sex drive, erectile dysfunction, poor body image, and orgasmic issues are all amendable to psychological and medical treatment. *True or false?*
6. Romantic intimacy, sexual ambivalence, and sensual touching are unrelated to each other. *True or false?*
7. Chronic use of pornography can become a mental health problem involving depression, anxiety, low self-worth, and increased isolation for men. *True or false?*
8. Sexual addiction is a minor addiction issue compared to others such as alcoholism, heroin, and cocaine. *True or false?*
9. Impotency (sexual performance) and lack of sexual intimacy (sexual desire) can be consciously and unconsciously impacted by prior abuse, bullying, mental health issues, parental views of sex, and religious perspective. *True or false?*
10. Birth control is the responsibility of the woman. *True or false?*
11. There is a difference between "fucking" and "making love." *True or false?*
12. Sexual fantasies should be kept to oneself because of their imaginary nature; fantasy is always better than real-life sexual partners and experiences. *True or false?*
13. Masculinity is not defined, formed, or developed by one's sexual orientation or preference. *True or false?*
14. Defining your masculinity based on the number of sexual partners you have had is a healthy sign of a balanced psychological sexual perspective. *True or false?*
15. Monogamy is an outdated puritanical belief that is no longer relevant or possible in marriage-type relationships. *True or false?*

How did you feel about these questions? We could complete ten pages of Q and A and only scratch the surface of this volatile subject—sex and men. For most men growing up, discussing sex was a nonstarter and, in fact, discouraged. The reality is that the majority of men are educated by a bunch of their fifteen-year-old buddies, telling each other about the dynamics of male-female male-male sex, female orgasms, how women get pregnant, and relationships. Sexual wisdom isn't passed along by teenage boys then, today, or throughout history. The dynamics of sex that go beyond erections, climaxing, feelings generated by sexual connections, and intimate, loving relationships were not part of our discussions growing up.

Clearly these boys—and I am included—had a limited knowledge base to draw from, coupled with no experience and understanding of ourselves or women—hence the rise in pornography viewing. In my psychological practice during the last thirty years, I have found that it's a challenge for men to be completely transparent about their sexual concerns, desires, cravings, fears, and failed and successful experiences. The taboo nature of sex is something we directly address for the sake of not furthering the knowledge gap for men. The ongoing discussion of developing a fulfilling sexual partnership with our partner is a relevant subject for men at any age.

Sexual orientation, bisexuality, homosexuality, and heterosexuality are some of the most heated personally and socially charged issues in our culture. Still, in many places around the world, it is a crime against the state to be gay or be involved in nonheterosexual relationship.

These questions and your answers are valuable for you to further understand who you are sexually. Accepting your sexual personality results in higher levels of satisfaction, contentment, and emotional fulfillment in all areas of our lives.

Finally, you may not agree with my answers nor do you need to—this is about you knowing you. The purpose is to widen our masculine perspective of healthy, mindful, emotionally balanced sexual behavior, sexual needs/cravings, sensuality, romance, and the role that sexual and personal awareness plays in our everyday life.

SEXUAL ANSWERS AND IDEAS FOR EXPANDING MASCULINE UNDERSTANDING

1. Sexual identity is a fixed issue, a permanent character quality and behavior for a man's entire life: *False*. Psychology research shows that as men (and women) develop, mature, and discover new things about themselves, their

sexuality also evolves. A deeper appreciation of who you are, expressing yourself in a completely vulnerable way, is emotionally liberating and healing. A man's starting point sexually doesn't imply it is an ending point. Rather, the experience of complete trust and psychological release is part of the masculine journey.

2. Sexual performance is different than sexual desire: *True*. Sexual desire for your partner can increase over a lifetime and during the course of the relationship. Sexual performance is directly connected to your physical body, health, age, drug use, sleep, testosterone levels, and chronic pain medications. Men generally judge their manhood by their sexual performance, which is *not* related to their sexual desire. Desire and performance are independent of one another—they are different sides of the same coin. Many times, sexual performance and sexual desire can be a great combination, but when they aren't, it is critical to understand the issues mentioned above. As men age, their sexual performance can be negatively impacted and their sexual desire can increase.

3. Women enjoy sex less than men: *False*. This is an old myth. In fact, as women age, their sexual desire and body acceptance increases along with their freedom to express their sexuality. Finding a partner with a mutual sexual desire, craving, and style is a fantastic benefit of intimate relationships. Men embracing their sexual desire tend to focus on shared intimacy rather than their orgasm. The emotional bonding that occurs with a sexual meeting of the hearts is transformational for both parties. Sexuality is much more than a physical release; it is a complete inner personal experience.

4. Homosexuality is a mental disorder created by an overbearing maternal figure or absent father figure in a young boy's life: *False*. The psychology of homosexuality has evolved dramatically during the last fifty years in the Western world. Homosexuality is no longer a mental illness, personality disorder, emotional flaw, or damaged boy. The relationship between biology and sexual orientation is an ongoing topic in psychology. Science doesn't fully understand how sexual orientation is caused or created. The argument of nature versus nurture is an endless debate. Being openly gay in many parts of the country and world is dangerous and not advisable. *Sexual orientation does not determine a man's masculine development but is a factor of his sexual expression.* The resistance historically by men to anything except heterosexuality is the driving force behind sexual prejudice—the fear of men loving men. Homophobia is a common term for sexual prejudice and discrimination for a peron's sexual preference. Mate

selection and all the factors involved is discussed later in part II, "Relationships Matter."

5. Low sex drive, erectile dysfunction, poor body image, and orgasmic issues are all amendable to psychological and medical treatment: *True*. Many times when men enter their thirties and forties, their body chemistry is impacted by aging, stress, lifestyle habits, or long-term alcohol or drug use, which negatively impacts sexual function. Sexuality is the combination of a man's preference, desire, performance, and attitude toward his sexual partner. The vast majority of sexual dysfunctions are amenable to many types of treatments; medical, psychological, medications, and so forth. The good news—as we discussed earlier—is that men are highly motivated to address their sexual problems immediately rather than someday. Oftentimes, underlying health issues can be treated with a proactive attitude. Men will not allow their "broken penis" to go unnoticed or avoid the reasons for its dysfunction.

6. Romantic intimacy, sexual ambivalence, and sensual touching are unrelated to each other: *False*. Emotional intimacy, vulnerability, and complete psychological transparency with your sexual partner is the fabric of a fulfilling sex life. Resistence and avoidance to being emotionally open, making eye contact, and hugging before and after sex are all critical elements for building a foundation of intimacy in your life. Men crave to be deeply understood, and sexual intimacy is a direct pathway to the meaningful parts of one's life. The unresolved traumas, emotional blocks to intimacy, and internal psychological rules for sex can be a man's worst enemy if left unexamined. Sex, intimacy, hugging, and being honest all require one primary element: vulnerability.

7. Chronic use of pornography can become a mental health problem involving depression, anxiety, low self-worth, and increased isolation for men: *True*. Psychologists argue that chronic use of pornography can lead to severe mental health problems that can create a downward spiral of shame (self-hatred), depression, anxiety, and hopelessness. Seeking comfort via friendships has a marked different outcome for men than seeking comfort via pornography. Since the worldwide COVID-19 shutdown in 2020 and 2021, pornography is now considered the new drug for isolation, despair, and fractured relationships. These findings are researched based, not morally driven nor from a religious perspective. Habitual use of pornography is not a relationship substitution or a guide for sexual intimacy.

8. Sexual addiction is a minor addiction issue compared to others such as alcoholism, heroin, and cocaine: *False*. Sexual addiction is a real crisis,

not a made-up alibi for impulsive male sexual behavior. Sexual addiction involves behaviors and activities that include masturbation, phone sex, cybersex, and pornography—the problem with all addictions including sex is when you are consumed by these actions. Your sexual thoughts, sexual fantasies, sexual urges, and sexual activities can't be controlled and are all consuming. These activities cause distress, harm your health, your relationships, your career, and every other aspect of your life. Finally, the secrecy of these sexual actions becomes a man's relentless burden to emotionally unload but to no avail.

9. Impotency (sexual performance) and lack of sexual intimacy (sexual desire) can be consciously and unconsciously impacted by prior abuse, bullying, mental health issues, parental views of sex, and religious perspective: *True.* Sex includes the complete person; nothing is left out or avoided psychologically. The impact of unresolved childhood traumas for boys can show up in their adult sexual relationships as low desire, sexual identity confusion, erectile dysfunction, and sexual ambivalence. These behaviors (with no medical cause or injury) and many others impact our sexual performance and sexual desire. If a man doesn't feel emotionally or physically safe with his partner, his body will betray him. Many times, the inability to achieve erection is an emotional barometer of mental health concerns that might need to be addressed in the relationship. The role of anxiety, psychological problems, fear of being emotionally suffocated, fear of commitment, pregnancy, and infidelity are variables that impact a man's sexual performance, desire, and satisfaction. The inner play of our humanity and sexual expression is all connected and can't be compartmentalized long term. Our body keeps the score even when we consciously forget.

10. Birth control is the responsibility of the woman: *False.* This belief is more prevalent than most would think, myself included. Men of all ages tend to default to the old male myth that birth control is only a woman's responsibility. The responsibility for having sex is mutual, yet it is the woman's role to take care of the birth control. Therefore, men don't need to be involved with the discussion about contraception. Men are involved in this discussion, and it's a joint dialogue. For instance, wearing a condom, or "rubber," is for more than prevention of sexually transmitted diseases, but being sexually responsible. I remind men that the US government views your role in a baby's conception as a minimum eighteen-year responsibility. Always ask questions and be proactive with any sexual partner for everyone's safety and health.

11. There is a difference between "fucking" and "making love": *True*. There are unlimited ways to kiss, share oral sex, have sexual intercourse, and to be orgasmic. The term "fucking" denotes a passionate, rough, loud, "hot," and non-intimate or intimate sexual encounter. This type of sexual connection is all about the super-sensual moment for the passion-driven couple. Making love, on the other hand, is a much slower pace, with foreplay, tender touching, talking, emotional awareness of yourself and partner, and intimate vulnerable exchange. The goal is emotional connection inside and out with your partner. The passion-driven moment is all about the orgasm and having sexual fun. Neither style is better than the other. It is great for couples to explore a variety of sexual styles. It's important to note that having a "quickie" without the emotional bond with a partner can circumvent your ability to enjoy the transformative power of intimacy, love, and feeling understood. Many men prefer the "quickie fucking" to avoid the emotional closeness.

12. Sexual fantasies should be kept to oneself because of their imaginary nature; fantasy is always better than real-life sexual partners and experiences: *False*. The opportunity to trust one's deepest fantasies, wishes, desires, and sexual habits with a partner is truly intimate and emotionally and psychologically bonding. The courage to share our deepest secrets with our intimate partner continues to build a solid relational foundation. *No one is more vulnerable than with their emotional walls down during an intimate moment*. The taboos surrounding fantasy are when there is a lack of emotional structure or history to support the deepest level of transparency between a man and his partner. Domination, submission, and many other fantasies are important to share with your partner for the intrinsic bond that is developed. Relationships evolve over time and the sexual component must be considered in this process.

13. Masculinity is not defined, formed, or developed by one's sexual orientation or preference: *True*. Masculinity is defined by the qualities of compassion, empathy, personal responsibility, and having a direction in life. Our sexual orientation is the frame around the picture of our life. Gay men, bisexual men, and heterosexual men all must develop these inner character qualities in order to live a fulfilling life. The absence or lack of development of these core character qualities is the crisis facing men currently. Prejudice and discrimination due to sexual orientation is based in fear and a lack of understanding of the masculine journey. I discuss later in the book some of the goals and purposes that each man must resolve on his masculine path.

14. Defining your masculinity based on the number of sexual partners you have had is a healthy sign of a balanced psychological sexual perspective: *False*. The key—whether a man has one partner or fifty-two different partners a year—is based on his emotional and psychological ability to form and sustain relationships. Having numerous sexual partners doesn't necessarily mean a man is relationship phobic. The same holds true for the man who isolates himself at work and avoids any type of significant emotional contact with a woman—personal, professional, or socially. Masculinity and mental health are not measured by sexual partners but rather the motivation and intention behind these behaviors. *Intimacy requires courage*. Chronic avoidance of developing significant emotional bonds is problematic for men and their long-term mental and physical health. Men who have a significant romantic relationship live longer than their peers who skip those emotional connections. Mental health and healthy masculinity are measured by the ability to develop (we all can do this) significant relationships!

15. Monogamy is an outdated puritanical belief that is no longer relevant or possible in marriage-type relationships: *False*. If sex is one of the hottest topics on the planet, then monogamy, faithfulness, and infidelity are its cousins. The topic is part and parcel to many men avoiding romantic commitment, fathering-parenting commitments, and developing secure relationship with a partner. The fear of being emotionally "suffocated" by a partner is one of the unspoken reasons men sidestep exclusive romantic relationships. As are all things in a relationship, monogamy is a choice. Men who choose faithfulness with their partner rather than defaulting into monogamy tend not to struggle or want to jump ship from their partner. Defaulting into a commitment is usually based in the fear of losing your partner and not fully giving yourself emotionally to the relationship. Men who avail themselves to the evolving process of sexual growth, discovery, and trust with their partner do not have the emotional need for a "filler" or escape exit. Commitment requires ongoing effort, time, energy, forgiveness, understanding, and desire to be a partnership. Monogamy is a by-product of these choices a man makes. We explore this topic and commitment issues for men in part II, "Relationships Matter."

QUESTIONS ABOUT YOU

- What is one topic, issue, or thought you had while reading and answering these questions?

- What is something about your sex life or sexuality you would like to address, explore, or discuss with your partner?
- How important is sex in your relationship(s)?
- Are you content with your sex life?

These four questions are the types of questions that I want you to start considering, asking yourself, asking your partner, and discussing with your close friends. Transparency with our inner circle of friends and partner organically builds and strengthens our inner self and sense of self-acceptance. Shame, depression, and anxiety can't thrive or exist when we expose our deepest fears and self-doubts.

CONNOR'S STORY—I ALWAYS KNEW!

From the beginning of preschool, Connor knew he liked boys differently than girls. He enjoyed being around girls at school and in the neighborhood, yet Connor always had an emotional pull toward certain boys he knew. During high school, Connor took girls to school dances and hung out with them but had an ever-growing emotional connection to men. Finally in his sophomore year of college, Connor, with great anticipatory anxiety, decided to tell his father that he was gay. His dad owned a construction company, according to Connor, and his father wasn't emotionally expressive or psychologically insightful. When Connor came out to his father, his dad smiled and said, "I was wondering when you were going tell me and your mother!" Connor found his father's response comforting and supportive; what he had feared didn't happen: rejection and disownment by his family. Connor's mother was also supportive of him becoming the best version of himself, regardless of his sexual orientation. Today, fourteen years later, Connor is a man in his mid-thirties who struggles with intimacy issues and fears feeling defective or not good enough. Connor first came to see me regarding a breakup with the "love of his life" whom he dated on and off for six years. His ex-partner wanted to settle down, get married, and have or adopt a baby. Connor was not interested or ready because his real-estate development company needed all of his energy and effort.

Connor and I discussed in therapy his reluctance to being vulnerable or feeling exposed if he fully committed to his partner. Connor believed that if he completely opened his heart to his partner, his partner would leave him— clearly irrational, coupled with a visceral feeling of inadequacy. Contrary to

Connor's fear, his partner had been loyal and faithful to him their entire relationship. The issue of not feeling like a man and not feeling good enough or capable enough were the hidden roadblocks that held Connor back. The years spent feeling defective for his sexual orientation has left Connor with a distorted view of his value in relationships and to himself.

The choice to resolve these outdated irrational beliefs, to be intimately courageous, and to move forward was causing Connor extreme sadness and shame—feelings of being unworthy of love. Connor's struggle with commitment, intimacy, and vulnerability is not a sexual orientation issue but rather personal growth relationship challenges.

AN ONGOING DEFINITION OF MASCULINITY—WHAT IS A MAN?

Human sexuality is not always about being labeled. It's about having a human moment, an emotion.—Cheo Hodari Coker

This quote is a great launching point for our ongoing male sexuality dialogue. Masculinity is a developmental experience, process, and learning curve that continues through puberty, into our earlier twenties, and leveling out later in life—but never stopping. Young men don't fall into or flip the switch on for manhood. Masculinity is developed as part of a man's core self throughout his entire lifetime—it's not a quick weekend course. Masculinity is central part of the core identity of who and what a man is becoming and will continue to become until he passes on.

The development of the four internal qualities that encompass our body, emotions, relationships, and psychological self is a fluid process, not a destination. After discussing sex, sexual intimacy, performance, and sexual orientation, it is time to give some more substance to this vague yet palpable topic all men know: what's healthy masculinity and men's mental health?

Professionally and personally speaking, most men can't articulate what a positive masculine man is. Men know what negative, abusive, and toxic self-centered masculinity looks, feels, and acts like. For our purposes, I have deliberately held off from defining masculinity, but rather outline the ideas with some white chalk on the ground where your cement foundation will be poured and built upon in the following chapters. You hold the blueprints for how you want your life to be built in the future.

Being unapologetically masculine isn't toxic. Know what you want and pursue it. Be assertive. Don't settle. Develop a deep self-worth. Learn to navigate your own emotions so others aren't responsible for them. And be kind. This requires the courage that defines masculinity.—Conner Beaton

This quote by Mr. Beaton is timeless, accurate, and hits men in the heart of the matter. Reread this quote and consider the ways in which you might want to become a better man. I discuss how to accomplish and implement this new masculinity model later in the book.

It's important, perhaps vital, that as a group of men we get away from the notion that if you are not a 110 percent heterosexual, meat-eating, cigar-smoking, womanizing billionaire, then somehow you have fallen short as a man. This may sound extreme and dramatic, but it is not. Courage to swim against the traditional male "nonfeeling" paradigm is necessary.

Unfortunately, the outdated tough-guy image is still culturally prevalent as much as smartphones are for young adults. It's an unspoken and ever-present measuring stick that most men feel beaten up by. Young men look to older men for guidance on how to be a man.

Both ends of the male masculinity continuum offers limited emotional insight for self or others or appropriate means for expressing their feelings or frustration tolerance. Some of the painful extremes for the masculine spectrum are a lack of emotional intelligence, poor problem-solving skills, aggressive or passive communication skills, and the inability to understand consequences. Each extreme suffers from its own form of rage, isolation, and hopelessness. Neither type of man is content or at peace with his life and its current status. Having a balanced masculinity is where a man will find his fulfillment, value, meaningful relationships, psychological stability, life purpose, mental health, and sense of belonging.

The quality of our life is directly linked to the healthiness of our relationship with ourself and others.—Joann Travis

Four Parts of the Masculine Definition

The four cornerstones to developing a healthy sense of your maleness start with understanding the intrinsic short-term and long-term value of these four interrelated qualities. Each quality is separate and related to the other four:

Compassion is the ability to accept yourself; embracing the areas of your life that are painful, feel shameful, and are not your best qualities per your own perspective. Your sense of self-compassion is the result of addressing, exposing, and healing your trauma(s); accepting your life journey as your own choice; and not blaming others for your past. You have the understanding and capacity to accept your childhood, family, partner, and the events that have been traumatic, painful, or abusive in your past; you accept, forgive, and understand yourself for things you can control and things you can't control.

Empathy is a byproduct of self-acceptance, which allows you to feel, understand, and psychologically acknowledge what someone else is going through. You are aware of how your actions and choices can impact others; you know how to respond to others without reacting to others' behaviors as personal attacks. You have a sense of yourself and the ability to form emotional boundaries in your relationships. You feel someone's struggle without becoming that person or responsible for them.

Life plan: You have the desire, emotional courage, and the psychological tenacity to consider, develop, and follow a plan for living your life personally, relationally, professionally, and physically. You have goals and find purpose in living your life; you are willing to take risks and follow your dreams to find your fulfillment.

Belief in yourself and something bigger than you: You humbly believe in yourself and that your life is purposeful; you know that your life is part of something bigger than your own self-interest and goals. You sense a higher self—your life has a purpose and meaning—and a collective consciousness in which we are all connected and matter. Your best (healed) self has meaningful purpose, and what you do matters now and in the future.

SUMMARY—KEEPING YOUR BALANCE

These four components are the foundational corners or building blocks to your masculine journey and mental health healing. Each of these facets of your masculinity is independent, interdependent, and interconnected with the others. This is an ongoing process of expanding your personal awareness of others, removing your denial of your past heartbreaks and losses, and achieving emotional stability in your life in these areas. How you express and implement passion and empathy in your life is your own opportunity, plan, and purpose. It's impossible to be an abusive man with a sense of empathy for others, because your abusive actions would be injurious to yourself. It's impossible to blame your partner for your lack of career advancement when you take full responsibility for your life goals, plan, and purpose. Arrogance and self-centeredness can't exist when you understand that your life is bigger than your immediate world.

> *The secret of change is to focus all of your energy, not on fighting the old, but on building the new.*—Socrates

Building a life with and around these four elements of a healthy, balanced, and psychologically healed man is exciting to be a part of. I continue to expand on these four elements of modern masculinity and how they relate to the mind-body connection, emotional intelligence, relationships, and your personal and best self. The key, as so eloquently stated by Socrates, is to focus your energy and actions on evolving as a man, not resenting your manhood or past.

CHAPTER FOUR

MASCULINITY AND YOUR BODY

Mind, Body, and Psychological Connections

Your body hears everything your mind says!—Annelie Howling

Those who do not find time for exercise will have to find time for illness.—Edward Smith-Stanley

These two quotes are timeless and telling of the intrinsic connection between our bodies, minds, and emotions—ultimately, everything is connected. Gentlemen, there is no avoiding this ever-increasing masculine awareness that the sum of the parts (your entire body, mind, soul) is greater than the whole (you)! This may sound counterintuitive, but it isn't. Embracing, accepting, and learning about all the parts of your medical well-being, mental health process, emotional cycles, relationship desires, and personal well-being is the road map for living a fulfilled life, which has a positive impact now and for generations to come.

The alternative to developing your masculine self is the isolation and avoidance of these parts of yourself! Avoidance leads to isolation and then to hopelessness—this is the male danger zone. Men don't thrive and can't exist for long periods of time in this negative, self-rejecting cycle of shame. Avoiding our feelings, denying our past, and isolating create our private "hell," in which we are terrorized by shame. *Isolation from ourselves and others is the single greatest threat to our mental health, our lives, our health, our relationships, our careers, our finances, and our lives.* Isolation and loneliness is a ticking time bomb that kills men of all ages—literally and figuratively! These elements combine in so many of the self-destructive examples of men who commit violent crimes against themselves (suicide); against their families, in mass shootings, and with emotional-physical terrorism. Let's now focus on how to heal our isolation by starting with some basic insights into our daily life.

We covered a lot of territory in the first part of our journey together. We discuss some of the more common issues facing men in this chapter and throughout the book, including

- Food issues: eating disorders (men really do have them)
- Alcohol, smoking, and recreational drugs: their long-term physical impact
- Vanity: male body dysmorphia, hair loss, aging
- Adonis complex (obsessive bodybuilding): muscle loss and weight gain
- Urology: prostate cancer; physical aging, and testosterone
- Medication usage: when and why mood stabilizers are valuable
- Surgery: knee, hip, heart, eye, and shoulder

Men's masculine thought: Only 30 percent of a man's health is determined by genetics; the other 70 percent is determined by his lifestyle (i.e., choices).

Naturally occurring, unavoidable physical issues impact your mental and emotional health, all of which is linked to how you live your life. Your physical evolution has psychological ramifications that seem daunting and scary—but are they really?

Removing the mud from our core self results in clarity about our personal issues. Think of this analogy: we have a gold brick at our core inner self. From our early years through young adulthood, our gold brick becomes covered with the mud of fear and ambivalence about our circumstances and traumas. The ability to wash off the mud shame starts with embracing these stages. Your body, emotions, relationships, and core self are all part of this personal experience, which is necessary to complete a 360-degree balanced life. The alternative is arrested emotional, psychological, and intellectual development.

Men's masculine thought— Embracing all the phases of your life is the formula for maximizing your career, emotional health, and relationships.

Most men die between the ages of twenty to twenty-seven but won't be buried until their 80s!—Unknown

The process of growing up is universal, and the expression of these steps becomes our personality—individuality. The onset of mental illness developmentally delays steps toward individuality. These delays fragment a man's inner sense of himself and distort his world view rather than creating a positive picture within of himself. The inner mirror a man creates of himself starts with how he sees and experiences trust, autonomy, independence, mastery, individuality, and the ongoing process called being a "man."

All our choices matter! Our physical, mental, emotional, family, romantic, sexual, career, and lifestyle choices impact the quality of our life more than we might believe or know. Seventy percent of our life is directly impacted by the choices we make; this includes our body choices, what we eat, our sleep habits, sexual

Men's masculine thought: Our mental health is directly impacted by positive health choices or negligent health choices— it's our choice every day!

expression, exercise, weight gain/loss, recreation, and whom we marry.

Accepting the responsibility of our choices is the only way to learn the lessons embedded in these seemingly disappointing, heartbreaking, and often-times traumatic experiences in our past.

- What is something you are willing to change about your health?
- What is something you are avoiding or postponing making a decision about regarding your lifestyle?
- What is one quality/part of your health, appearance, or body that you like?
- What is a physical issue you have to manage?

These questions are a sampling of the vast array of choices you can make to change your present-day life. Fear of making a mistake or making the wrong choice is a myth. All your actions are choices; even when you don't take action, that is a choice. The personal power of accepting responsibility for your choices is the fast lane to experiencing fulfillment that can't

Choice breeds responsibility; responsibility breeds fulfillment; fulfillment breeds balanced masculine mental health!

be bought or acquired with money. No one can take it away unless you give it away! More on this topic of male placating/people-pleasing habits in part II, "Relationships Matter." We now step into the rushing river of food, personal appearance, and why it matters for men.

FOOD, MEN, AND THE PERFECT APPEARANCE

A question I am asked frequently regarding weight loss and food is, "Do I have an eating disorder?" My first thought is, *Why are you asking this question?*

Usually, my clients ask because they know intuitively that something isn't right or that their body image issues are out of balance. Then we discuss the definition of eating disorders according to the psychological bible of mental health and mental illness disorders, the *Diagnostic and Statistical Manual of Mental Disorders* (DSM-5): "Feeding and eating disorders are characterized by a persistent disturbance of eating or eating related behavior that results in the altered consumption or absorption of food and that significantly impairs physical health or psychological functioning" (329).

If an eating disorder is left unchecked, it can lead to serious mental and physical health crises, even premature death. According to the DSM-5, the common factors and behaviors that manifest in eating issues include, but are not limited to, the following:

- Restricted caloric intake leading to significant weight loss—below accepted medical levels for your height, body type, and age
- Medically "dangerous" weight loss for the age and body of the man
- Intense fear of gaining weight or becoming "fat"
- Daily life is centered around the obsession with food, calories, and imaginary weight gains
- Lack of understanding about the medical dangers an eating behavior is causing or can cause the individual—no insight into the cycle of weight gain
- Lack of acknowledgment of the seriousness of a "skinny" appearance and the declining health associated with one's food, weight, calorie-counting obsession
- Uncontrollable impulse to gorge/binge, overeating to the point of becoming physically sick
- Misuse of laxatives, diuretics, or enemas as a means to control imaginary weight gain; ignoring the serious health risks associated with abuse of these over-the-counter medicines
- Damage to the gums and teeth as a result of binging/purging cycle for extreme weight loss. Stomach acid from repeated vomiting damages the throat, teeth, and gums. Long-term vomiting can cause esophageal cancer.
- The food/body/weight obsession causes significant psychological distress, anxiety, despair, delusional thinking, and, in severe cases, thoughts of suicide. The man's life is preoccupied with food, weight gain/loss, and physical appearance.
- Prolonged maladaptive eating such as binging/purging negatively impacts the body's brain chemistry, causing a lack of production of the four primary neurotransmitters—serotonin, dopamine, oxytocin, and endorphins.

Our brains depend on these chemicals for optimal functioning. Our mental health depends on our brain function, and these chemicals are essential for balanced mental, physical, relational, and personal functioning.

YOU, YOUR FOOD CHOICES, AND YOUR BODY: A QUESTIONNAIRE

Be completely honest about your relationship to food, your body, and your mental well-being. The food you eat affects your body and mind, and eating is a natural experience that can't be disregarded. You can live without drinking wine, doing drugs, and smoking marijuana, but you can't live without eating! This is why your relationship to food, your health, your appearance, and your emotions are connected and complicated. Answer the following questions with your first thought—no editing your answers.

- How many of these clinical behaviors, actions, or descriptions apply to you?
- How many times have you gone on a diet and why?
- How often do you use food to self-soothe?
- Do you like your body and appearance?
- Do you exercise for health or to look good?
- How important is food in your daily life and in your relationships?
- Do people comment on your appearance in a positive or negative manner?
- Are you secretly scared of being overweight or too thin?
- Does your appearance impact your mood?
- Do you have good dental habits?
- Do you substitute drinking or smoking for eating?
- How comfortable are you with your current appearance and weight?
- How much of your sense of "masculinity" is attached to your appearance?

This is a brief overview of the potential pitfalls of eating, weight loss, and their interaction with our mental health and outlook on life. Reread the clinical definitions of eating issues if you are worried about your private thoughts or secrets about you and your body. Male eating disorders are serious. It's important to know that all food-related psychological and physical issues are treatable with great outcomes. Suffering in silence is no

Men's masculine thought—25 percent of males with normal weight perceive themselves to be overweight, according to the National Eating Disorders Association

longer a choice that you need to make! Your entire life is impacted by your body and food relationship.

There will never be an area of your life that isn't impacted by your relationship to food, weight gain/loss, or body image concerns. How you view your body is an essential element of compassion for yourself and empathy for others.

Looking like a man—whatever that means—is part and parcel to the old-school male myth of masculinity. This narrow perspective of men is still prevalent, influencing men of all ages and walks of life: what must a man look like?

As discussed earlier in the book, it is time for young, middle-aged, and older men to embrace their body type and appearance. My professional experience is that younger men, particularly, lack the support and understanding to "unpack" their concerns, fears, and negative self-talk about their appearance, body, and athletic ability. The pressure from social media, sports ads, beer commercials, and media advertisements with the perfect-looking, jacked-up guy is everywhere. What does the ideal man look like? The $10 million question of the day: can a mentally balanced man have fulfilling relationships, a career, be slim, unathletic, shy, average looking, and masculine?

Yes, and yes again. The updated version of masculinity we discuss here isn't based on a man's physicality, appearance, or some arbitrary fashion trend. Appearance is a personal matter, regardless of how pop culture pressures men to conform.

The emotional fallout for body image issues—poor health, chronic illness, fat-shaming, self-loathing—are mental health challenges. The medical community is keenly aware that a man's emotional struggles, spoken or unspoken, and feelings of hopelessness weaken his immune system and overall quality of life. The interplay of emotions and physical sickness is gaining more relevance as a psychosomatic issue. Health is no longer viewed as an isolated compartment of a man's life, but rather as a continuous circle of connections.

MENTAL HEALTH SUMMARY—WHEN DO I GET HELP?

Suggestions for Improving Our Overall Life

When should I get medication or see a mental health professional? Mood swings are natural and common to a point. When a negative or extremely expansive positive mood lasts for longer and longer periods of time, this could be a sign that you might be developing a low-level functional bipolar depression. The frequency and intensity of your negative and positive mood swings are valuable barometers for the stability of your psychological and physical chemistry. When you feel flat, without energy, as if everything takes an effort, stop showering, miss work, cancel social activities, isolate, and feel pessimistic about your life—these are red flashing lights. These warning signs alert you to the possible problems ahead concerning your mental stability and emotional health. At this point, or under similar circumstances, you could greatly benefit from some professional support—medical or psychological. Denial or avoiding these symptoms doesn't lessen or eliminate them. Without seeking treatment, these symptoms only increase in intensity and duration—read that again! *Something to ponder: cancer doesn't go into remission on its own, nor do mental health and psychological problems without treatment!* Seeking professional help is courageous positive masculinity, a mature and responsible choice.

Therapy is for the mentally ill; I am just sad, and I can work it out. Critical mood swings, sadness, hopelessness, despair, disappointment, panic, and fear of the future/impending doom are all emotional states that can be short-lived or increase with frequency and duration. It's a good rule of thumb that when you can't seem to shake off these feelings, then it is time to consider a medical/ mental health professional. Consulting with your medical doctor about your emotional state is as important as consulting with them about blood in your urine—it's imperative. Ignoring your mental and physical health would never happen if your penis was falling off. Yet we men (me included) put our head in the sand (or someplace else), minimizing these glaring problems. Your partner or a close friend can be a valuable source of information about your emotional struggles. The people closest to you are incredible sources of information, insight, and support, if you question the validity of your current psychological and physical condition. Just ask them and they will be very relieved that you are open-minded about addressing your physical and mental health issues. Avoidance breeds everything we truly don't want in our lives—despair!

I can work out at the gym, and my problems are under control—my partner can be my therapist. Make no mistake, working out is great, a fabulous source of pure energy and mental boost. Unresolved emotional traumas such as your divorce, an ongoing child custody fight, an affair, job loss, a teenager's drug issues, depression, lingering guilt, shame, and feelings of unworthiness can't be addressed, healed, or resolved with obsessive exercising. In fact, the hyperfocus on the body to the exclusion of your mental health creates emotional emptiness. For instance, the Adonis complex is the overemphasis on muscular development. Men who get caught up in the bodybuilding craze, body worship, body dysmorphia, eating disorders cycle, and excessive training programs believe that their bodies are their lives. Our bodies are part of our lives, but they don't define or address our mental, relational, and emotional health challenges—we do!

Your partner doesn't want to be your mental health counselor, therapist, or mother! If he or she does, that's another set of problems for the relationship section. We all need a neutral, professionally trained psychologist or therapist to properly diagnose and teach us how to heal ourselves. Therapy is about creating a new dialogue within and gaining new tools for our journey. These tools are coming in the following chapters.

I am always stressed, getting colds, and never enough sleep because of my job, family and responsibilities; I don't have time for all your self-care ideas. These are all legitimate concerns and understandable energy outputs. Consider the idea that your body is like a cell phone battery that only holds a charge so long until it is out of energy and no longer works. This holds true for our entire physical, emotional, and mental life. One of the skills necessary for long-term growth is learning the fine art of maintaining your internal balance. Your internal balance dictates how you react and respond to the stressors coming at you. Regardless of your circumstances, your mental, emotional, and psychological health and perspective is the foundation on which your life rests. When your internal axis is off, you are off balance, and nothing is going to work well. Living our lives out of balance is the cause of so many health issues for men that we have discussed. We choose our chaos, and we choose our peace. Choose wisely.

CHAPTER FIVE

MASCULINITY *IS* EMOTIONAL INTELLIGENCE

What Am I Feeling?

Before I could manage my emotions, I had to accept my emotions. Before acceptance, I had to identify my emotions. Before identifying, I had to acknowledge my emotions. Before acknowledgement, I had to be honest with myself. And this took work.—Russell, age forty-four, sober and drug free for more than twenty years

Russell is handing us the road map to the process of developing our emotional and mental health, increased awareness, and vulnerability with our feelings. We are going to go straight to the heart of the matter of what mental, psychological, and emotional health looks like for men! All these intangible elements of your feelings, emotions, psychological process, and mental state of mind are part and parcel of your emotional intelligence—how you and I experience and react to our world.

Intellectual/cognitive intelligence is wonderful and supports the functioning of your emotional/psychological intelligence; both parts need each other to help complete your mental health–life balance. Your emotional intelligence is how you live, react, and respond; it directs all your relationships. Our life is a series of various relationships, including our romantic partner, childhood and present-day family, colleagues, friends, siblings, and everyone else. The more you understand your internal world of living, the more functional and fulfilling your entire life will be—it's that direct and simple.

Two quick questions before we start:

- What is emotionally upsetting to you?
- How would you describe it?

I ask these two questions because we all know to some extent what we are feeling. Our feelings—if we engage and acknowledge their impact on our health, our friendships, our career and colleagues, our family and in-laws, our partner, and ourselves—are one of the barometers for the quality of our life. If we dismiss our feelings and emotions as trivial, nonissues, needless, or worse, we bury them, and the short- and long-term outcome isn't good.

If our psychology is so important and valuable to every aspect of our well-being, why do we avoid it? Oftentimes the reason is that our psychological growth was interrupted, delayed, and impaired. These childhood circumstances result in us minimizing our feelings and emotions, as if they are of minor importance. Rather, the opposite is true: our entire life is impacted by our processing of daily events. The lack of emotional understanding over time results in us "going through the motions" of living. Our fathers and grandfathers were never encouraged to access their greatest and most valuable resources: the psychological experience of the emotional power of love, acceptance, and peace of mind. You can't buy these personal psychological forces; you have to live them! Feeling empty is one of the by-products of being emotionally stunted and cut off, unable to interact with people and ourselves.

The quote below is a new reality that men are beginning to understand: that their mental health and psychological challenges will eventually appear in their relationships, especially intimate and romantic relationships. The days of dismissing and avoiding our uncomfortable feelings, disappointments, and self-defeating beliefs about not needing anyone are gone. Women, romantic partners, your family, your children, and your friends expect men (you and me) to develop our emotional intelligence skills, which no generation of men have done or perhaps ever attempted.

Think about that: your grandfather, father, uncles, cousins, and buddies have never been asked to develop their masculinity with psychological balance and a functional mental health perspective. Women want a partner who has the psychological maturity, insight, and the ability to be vulnerable, supportive, and emotionally understand her and himself. This is the purpose of this chapter—explaining, guiding, and expanding our psychological mental health capacities. Ultimately, nothing in our life will sustain long-term improvement without our understanding of our psychological self.

What you haven't healed from in yourself will show up in your relationships.—Norma Garcia, therapist, Los Angeles, California

WHAT IS MY MENTAL HEALTH?

For our purposes, let's clarify the distinctions between our feelings, emotions, psychology, and mental health as they function independently, together simultaneously, and help to coordinate your interior life. All four parts are simultaneously interdependent and independent. Our overview sheds some light on the intricate interplay of our deepest thoughts, values, beliefs, emotions, and feelings that define who and what we are to ourselves. We (you) are going to uncover what is in the back closet in your life. This takes courage, which you already have engaged, or you would not be reading this book. Courage has a huge personal payoff, a deep sense of peace and accomplishment. The alternative of avoidance and anger creates an emotional state of hopelessness, which leads to terrible outcomes.

Your Four-Part Process

Your Feelings

Your feelings are your personal internal reactions, experiences about the events and circumstances in your life. What you are "feeling" is highly individual, personal, subjective, and informational about you. Only you know your feelings! No one can truly tell you how to feel or why you feel the way you do. This is your full responsibility and challenge. Understanding or dismissing them as unnecessary is a health risk both physically and mentally. You assign meaning and value to your feelings. What is one person's feelings of sadness can be another's feelings of joy. Feelings are temporary and can change immediately depending on you and what you are perceiving. Your feelings can short-circuit or overwhelm your preset limitations on grief, sadness, happiness, joy, fear, and heartbreak or disappointment. Feelings are temporary emotional states. Like the tides of the ocean, they can change instantly or every twelve hours. Your feelings are processed through your internal filters, beliefs, and values.

Feeling "stressed" is a common statement and research topic. Stress is a feeling with serious health implications. Untreated stressful feelings such as anxiety and depression are major factors leading to cardiac arrest, stroke, and high blood pressure. Stressful feelings cause our bodies to create stress hormones such as cortisol to help our bodies manage the emergency. It's impossible for anyone to sustain balanced health with chronic feelings of despair, panic, and hopelessness. Negative feelings wear down the body, immune system, cardiovascular functioning, and the ability to fight diseases. These are some of the critical facts that your feelings are part and parcel to your physical health.

Your Emotions

Your emotions are your everyday life experiences that you translate, give meaning to in your mind, and that define your life. Emotions activate your internalized psychological belief system (conscious and unconscious) for how you feel about the event, person, or situation. You can't separate your emotions from your feelings—they are interconnected. Your emotional response or re-action tends to be automatic responses to your circumstances—feelings. This rapid reaction gives the illusion that your feelings affect your emotions and thoughts, but it's quite the contrary. Emotional reactions are unconscious in nature and have grown with you throughout all your life experiences, traumas, and intellectual maturity.

Your physical responses also manifest the emotions that you experience; for example, your heart starts racing, your breathing becomes shallow, and your face suddenly flushes with heat when you mentally "flash" on your ex-partner. These are all emotional reactions that your body is experiencing and signaling to you. Your emotions translate your feelings for you. Emotional beliefs that depict your value responses are consistent, stable, long-term, enduring states of mind. You might not know, but you have conscious and unconscious "emotional guard-rails" that allow you to experience the dualities of living—happiness/sadness, joy/disappointment, excitement/boredom, pleasure/pain, anxiety/calm, depres-sion/hope, and many more. These guardrails can be very narrow or very wide with twenty-six lanes of traffic going east and west. Your emotional bandwidth is something you have control of whether you know it or assume otherwise. Men typically in the past have had a very narrow bandwidth with which to feel, to think, or to experience any emotional state of mind other than neutral.

For example, you are buying a new car and the finance people question your credit rating. You feel a sudden wave of embarrassment, your face feels hot, and a sense of shame floods you with feelings like "damaged goods," and "imposter." You think the bank is punishing you; you view the questions as a personal indictment about you and your worthiness rather than as a business transaction. *Your emotional beliefs guide how you experience and translate your feelings in that moment.* Your emotions are a window into your core beliefs (spoken and unspoken) about you and all the areas of your life—physical, mental, relational, and personal. The backbone to your emotional life is your psychological beliefs and values.

Your Psychology

Your psychology is the internal intellectual processing center of your beliefs and values system: how you perceive your experiences. It is the lens through which you view your life and then respond emotionally to your wife, your clients, family, physical aches and pains, losses, disappointments, and achievements. Your psychological lens, along with your emotional insight, translates, analyzes, and gives meaning to your feelings. Your "internal software" is on, 24/7, all moments of your day and night. It's impossible to avoid this ongoing dynamic in your life. Your psychological process is highly individualized for you to make sense of your personal and professional relationships and your disappointments and successes. Your psychological process began developing at birth and continues as long as you live. Your sense of internal stability is your psychological foundation. Your conscious and unconscious thoughts, feelings, and mood swings *all* originate from your psychological perspective. What you secretly think and feel about yourself, your interactions with others, and the beliefs you have about life can be better understood with your psychological awareness. Your psychological thinking becomes your emotional expression and interpretation of your life.

The example of buying a new car is viewed through your psychological lens. The different thoughts, emotions, and feelings about buying your new car are invaluable information about you, your values, your core image, and how you want the world to see you; for example, what kind of car you choose; what that car represents socially and personally; the status you feel by owning this car; the emotional courage of having your finances examined by a third party; and the personal power to buy a new car.

All of these elements—your psychological values, your emotional expression, your feeling process—are in motion, working in conjunction. Men and their relationship with cars are one of the enduring traits of a "man's man." Men use possessions to measure themselves against other men, and cars are one of the most common measurements. What does your car, truck, or any personal possession to which you attach personal meaning say about you?

Your Mental Health

Your mental health encompasses *all of you*: your emotional cycles, your interpretation of your mood and feelings, and how you frame and define your life situation is your ongoing psychology. All the elements of your feelings, emotions, perspectives, and psychological expressions comprise your mental health. How each element functions together and independently forms a picture of your overall mental health worldview. This includes what you value, desire, hope for, and fear. Your mental health is your public statement about how you feel and live every day of your life.

Mental Health Is the "Invisible" Body Containing All the Parts of You

For clarification purposes, let's use the analogy that your mental health is the CEO of your life. Its role is to oversee your psychological views, your emotional reactions, how you feel, which impacts your body, cognitive functioning, relationships, and perspective on your life. This enormous responsibility of your mental health encompasses, represents, directly controls, impacts, and directs every second of your life. Your mental health is the primary foundational element of your life. We all have this hardware, but do we nurture it, embrace it, accept it, or avoid it?

Now that we have a broader understanding of our mental health dynamic, it's time to dig below the busyness of our day and learn more about our inner workings. Let's explore some of the emotional roadblocks men experience when expressing their internal thoughts. My suspicion is that men get "freaked out"—overwhelmed—and shut down mentally when our emotional comfort level is overloaded. Any type of circumstance of intense verbal or nonverbal expression that triggers a knee-jerk reaction can be likened to sticking your finger into electric outlet and trying not to die.

Men learn at early age through peer pressure, bullying, and emotionally unavailable parental figures that strong emotional expression—other than anger—is unacceptable. Boys don't cry nor show their sadness, fear, or terror. Verbalizing, understanding, and expressing our internal thoughts and feelings is a developed skill set that requires unlearning the old "tough-guy" habits. The problem is that these boys grow up and become men in positions of influence in their families, jobs, and communities with little to no understanding of their own mental health.

EMOTIONAL GROWTH—REMOVING THE "MALE GAG ORDER"

The cave you fear to enter holds the treasure you seek!—Joseph Campbell, scholar

Now that we understand the interplay of our four-part mental health process, let's delve into the heart of why men choose silence over emotional connection. Ripping the bandage off your own emotional-verbal "gag order" is literally removing the blinders from your repressed psychological body. The opportunity to experience your own vulnerability without fear, terror, anger, rage, depression, and violence taps in to your inherent potential of contentment, fulfillment, and peace of mind. For a man to become the "guy" he wants to be, this deep dive into our inner cave is part of the natural process of healing, accepting, and discovering our "lost" pieces! The fragments and broken pieces of our childhood, teens, and current life must be individually picked up and reassembled into our complete psychological self.

Psychologically shutting down or numbing oneself to one's emotions starts as a safety reaction in childhood that evolved many, many years ago. The reasons for it are varied but ultimately in order to survive a chaotic family, unpredictable home circumstances, and terrifying physical and emotional events, compartmentalizing our feelings was the only way to grow up. Survival in childhood becomes an automatic psychological reaction to unsafe, dangerous, and neglectful parents. The idea of revisiting or doing an unguided archaeological dig into your childhood isn't the goal. Our sole purpose is to uncover, name, and eliminate your emotional triggers, psychological roadblocks, and unresolved trauma.

Our "man cave" is the place where we buried painful, unspeakable memories that still haunt us and control our lives today without our conscious awareness or consent. Think about that for a moment: what events or emotions do you avoid, dismiss, or ignore to avoid experiencing and acknowledging them? (Everyone has an answer for this.)

We (you and me) are going to enter your dark cave, where no man—not even you—has been allowed to enter. Our dark cave contains the unhealed, rageful parts of ourselves. This is why you are emotionally avoidant—psychological numb—to certain emotions. These early survival tools were developed on the fly and for valid reasons. The starting point to reclaiming your emotional health and reconnecting the fragmented pieces of yourself begins now!

Cautionary Note 1

We are not finger-pointing, blaming anyone, or fabricating problems about your past. Quite the contrary! This isn't a psychological exercise for becoming a self-pitying, self-absorbed, whiny man-child. Our purpose is to understand the circumstances, critical events, and family environment that you learned to psychologically survive and grow up in. We can't skip this step in our healing process—it provides the context of who you are and why. For instance, acknowledging that your childhood was crazy, chaotic, embarrassing, or depressing isn't self-indulgent. Acknowledging

Wisdom is understanding your family. Immaturity is blaming your family.

your past is very different than blaming your past and the people in it! One road leads to healing and the other leads to emotional hell.

Cautionary Note 2

When we get caught up in the "blame game"—and many men do—it creates more and more resentment. Resentment left to fester leads to extremely dangerous outcomes for you, your health, and your relationships. Resentment and blaming are purposeless, serving no value in understanding your psychological trauma. Regardless of your circumstances, blaming doesn't eliminate the abuse or heal you, so it is always a waste of your time. Blaming is like running around a track for years and wondering why you haven't made any progress in your life, in your relationships, and with your mental health.

Blaming is seductive, breeding emotional confusion while avoiding responsibility.

Blaming is the quickest way to avoid taking present-day responsibility and becoming proactive rather than reactive in our lives. Resenting and hating our fathers for not being the fathers we wanted or needed leads us down a dead-end street. Eventually we turn our life around or we die waiting for an apology that isn't coming and may never come!

Blaming and holding resentment is a form of emotional cancer that devours the accuser, not the person of blame. My goal and intention are to expand your psychological understanding of your emotional blocks and how you can work through them. Healed men are men who change their world and the world around them. I discuss in later chapters the different ways to release your resentments,

You can't let go of what you don't know you are holding! Until you know what it is or its control in your life, nothing is going to change for you—nothing!

to let go of your traumas, and to stop blaming your past while taking full responsibility and ownership of your life. You are ultimately setting yourself free from your past.

Where Things Started

Children don't know the difference between a crazy childhood and peaceful boring childhood. We just don't know that until later in life. Kids assume that every family is like theirs until around adolescence, when they begin comparing stories, which becomes eye opening. Repeated exposure to fear, anger, and violent events cause children to develop a psychological process of fight-or-flight emotional reaction for their physical and mental survival. Your family might have seemed normal on the outside but maybe things didn't feel safe or predictable inside the house.

Many years later, as an adult man, you witness your partner's volatile emotional response to something unrelated to you, which unconsciously activates your automatic fight-flight reaction to danger. This happens in the blink of eye (literally), and you instinctively shut down emotionally and mentally. This psychological, physical, and mental shutdown is impenetrable and never fails the user (you). Over time, your defense mechanism for surviving unsafe situations and circumstances, real or imagined, becomes unconscious, without any pause or psychological resistance on your part. The terror that a young boy buries to survive childhood is a primary reason men avoid their feelings, emotional expression, or anything that opens their mental health, which is a door bolted shut. When someone expresses strong "negative" emotions, it triggers the unconscious emotional cycle of fear, which breeds shame and self-blame. Negative emotions, which feel dangerous to this adult man, originate in his childhood. Unresolved emotional experiences, negative beliefs, and severe reactions of fear and anger are elements of unresolved trauma.

"Teacher, what does it mean to work on yourself?"
"It is to stop waiting for the others to change."—Chinese proverb

Our emotional capacity for engaging and understanding ourselves and other people is almost impossible when our psychological lenses are clouded with emotional despair. The layers and layers of emotional defenses against ever feeling vulnerable, powerless, and scared is complicated. The ability to stop—to understand your psychological superpower within—is a learned task.

This is the work of going to therapy, couples counseling, life coaches, and men's groups; for reading books like this; for meditating; and for journaling to uncover and heal our inner boy. Developing insight to manage our frustration, to express empathy, to feel disappointment, to accept love, to be forgiving, and to receive compliments or criticism is our emotional intelligence (EI) working at full potential! Think about your EI strengths and areas that need improvement, development, change, and understanding. The following questions are teasers for beginning to explore the buried pieces of you.

1. What is an incident, situation, or circumstance from your past that might be lingering and negatively impacting your present-day marriage, relationship, or parenting?

2. What is one of your emotional strengths?
3. What is emotionally difficulty for you?
4. Take a moment to think about an interaction or a recent conversation that caused you to feel emotionally uncomfortable or uneasy or that caused you to "lose your shit." Why did you react that way?
5. When you feel emotionally uncomfortable, is this an old pattern that you have had for many years or a new pattern? Why is it an old (or new) pattern?
6. What is one emotional fear or hesitation about your personal life that you fear someone else knowing?

Gentlemen, one of the requirements to living a fulfilling, purposeful life always includes being emotionally fluent with yourself and others. Embracing the "ugly" parts of our lives is the key to unlocking our greatest dreams and desires—hence being emotionally fluent. Your mental health healing process starts with an honest self-examination to gain clarity, not to increase your resentment. How did you answer the questions above? These types of insightful questions are for your self-discovery, for uncovering some of the lost emotional pieces of you. We don't want a skewed emotional life—out of balance, aggressive, or scary to us, our friends, and family. The inability to manage our anger outbursts—becoming verbally aggressive, physically violent, or unaware of our psychological triggers—is a warning sign that our unresolved emotional traumas are spilling into our day-to-day life.

I deal with women of all ages who continually try to convince me that their partners' violent outbursts are normal and what a man's man does! No and no again is my answer, with no apology about their denial concerning their psychological crisis. Scaring people, "losing your shit," pointing a gun at someone over a parking spot, or threatening to "kill" a partner who looks at another guy is insane and inexcusable. Dangerous overreactions and extreme threats of violence are the emotional ingredients of a male time bomb.

Sounds simple, but is it? Of course not! Discovering your emotional process and the need for health is as important as air to a drowning man.

Becoming the man you desire and knowing your "issues" requires personal courage to approach the unmentionable events in your past. We have to walk into our dark cave and open Pandora's box of hidden psychological "stuff." Your box of secrets isn't evil, as was the contents of Pandora's box in mythological Greek story. Rather, you're opening up and beginning your journey into manhood. Inside of you contains a map for accomplishing things you never considered or imagined to be possible.

The reward for our work is not what we get, but what we become.
—Paulo Coelho

Emotional Benefits of Confronting and Resolving Your Fears

First, your past isn't beyond healing or understanding. Our internal critics tell us we are damaged beyond repair—that's our shame and the next topic of discussion. Just know that unresolved shame is relentless, mercilessly causing us deep psychological and emotional terror—but is all within arm's reach of healing! Your self-imposed psychological limitations, emotional safety, shame, and dismissal of your painful experiences are devouring, blocking, and interfering with your ability to live your life today! The personal power and calmness that is gained by better understanding ourselves, our immediate circle of family, and friends without judgment or mistrust are possible.

Second, accepting and observing our feelings as informational—as a means of knowing about ourselves—is liberating. Freedom from your secrets and emotional terror is something only you can do.

Third, balanced emotional insight breeds improved physical, mental, and relational health. Experiencing positive emotions, thoughts, and feelings have been shown to be great antidotes to major diseases and mental illness. One of the most attractive qualities that women want in a man is one who can constructively engage with his emotions and hers. This man (you) has the "superpower" of insight and emotional awareness for any situation at work, at home, within family, or personally. Emotional intelligence breeds insight into yourself and others while increasing your new language skills—your emotional vulnerability.

MEN REJECTING THEIR FEELINGS—
STOPPING THE CYCLE OF EMOTIONAL IGNORANCE

Some of the most common emotionally terrifying, emasculating descriptions and destructive statements about men's emotional health come from other men; they are listed below. Men of the old masculinity model who are unable to emotionally connect, understand themselves, or be vulnerable use these types of statements to shut down any discussion of feelings. Unfortunately, men who express something other than anger end up being mocked, beaten, or alienated from the fraternity of men. Bullying is another way to prevent men from being open and honest.

Male "Nonstarter" Statements and Negative Beliefs

- Take it like a man.
- Real men don't show emotions.
- Man up!
- Keep it to yourself.
- Crying shows weakness.
- Boys cry; men don't cry.
- Women are too sensitive; don't be like that!
- Shake it off; you'll be fine; get over it!
- Don't be so emotional; get a grip on yourself; everyone dies.
- Dude, where's your backbone? It's no big deal; your girlfriend was a loser.
- Stop being so sensitive; you are scaring me.
- Don't be a pussy.
- Dude, you need medication.

How many of you have heard or been told these urban lies about men and their emotional expression? It's very painful for a young boy to experience the devastating humiliation by a parent for attempting to express their upset about something that happened at school earlier in the day. Or attempting to manage the terror of being bullied at work by coworkers. It's important to consider some counter-replies to these emotionally paralyzing male statements. These comments and others like them put a young man in an emotional straitjacket. This boy becomes an adult man with no idea of how to express or mange his or his partner's feelings. The majority of young and older men know that the current times are demanding higher levels of psychological insight and emotional awareness than what they developed or learned growing up. Listed below are some updated replies to "male silence" for men to psychologically push back their male counterparts.

Psychological Pushback against the Male Gag Order

- The new man has the masculine courage and the ability and aptitude to be emotionally fluent. High-functioning adult men express their feelings and manage their emotions in a responsible manner.
- Mature masculinity tolerates and manages negativity or rejection without responding angrily or violently.
- Choosing to be emotionally responsible with one's actions and words is very appealing to both men and women.
- Wisdom is the ability to discern who is and is not a personal confidant.

- Masculine courage includes the ability to celebrate and cry. Living between these two polarities of emotion is both challenging and rewarding.
- Suppressing, repressing, and denying my feelings isn't a choice I am willing to make. The emotional aptitude to express myself is a learned skill.
- Women want an equal partner—psychologically, emotionally, and mentally. Wealth is nice but it can't buy these traits.
- Avoiding, denying, and dismissing your past traumas only prolongs despair and emotional suffering. Confronting our issues is the only way out of the cycle of despair and loneliness.
- The past never stops living in the present until it is psychologically addressed. Unresolved emotional abuse, sexual abuse, rape, physical beatings, and any other traumatic experience don't disappear or vanish on their own. Emotional trauma resurfaces at the worst moments of your life. This unwelcome "trauma guest" negatively impacts your body and your health, distorts and destroys your relationships, blows up your career, sabotages your marriage, and scares and alienates your children.

Always do what you are afraid to do.—Ralph Waldo Emerson

Limited male emotional expression (other than anger) with other men might have seemed normal and felt safe in the past but not anymore. This belief wasn't true then or today. Denying one's emotional state can lead to serious psychological problems that can result in violent consequences for the individual and the community around him. Emotional expression among men builds strong psychological bonds that are invaluable for a man's mental and emotional health. Men need intimacy and the safety that comes with that inner security and relationship with other like-minded men. Emerson says to do what scares you: for us, that is to be emotionally vulnerable with ourselves and the people closest to us.

> *Emotional connection, insight, and understanding are the foundational elements for a fulfilling, committed, long-term relationship!*

SUMMARY THOUGHTS AND CONCLUSIONS— TWO MEN AND TWO CAUTIONARY TALES

Dr. Jonathan Guttman, a psychologist and expert on marriage and relationships, researched why women sought divorces. *Guttman discovered that 70 percent of the marriages that ended in divorce had a common theme: emotionally unavailable men.* The women reported that their partner was unable, unwilling, or didn't see the value in developing their emotional relationship. The man's resistance to and denial and neglect of emotional intimacy led to the marriage's demise.

Emotional vulnerability and connection are absolutely vital for a successful marriage or any other type of intimate relationship. The men who develop emotional intimacy and psychological vulnerability with their partners report the highest levels of marital satisfaction. The other 30 percent of the divorces in Guttman's study were unresolvable issues with many different variables, including violence, domestic abuse, drug use, infidelity, and money concerns.

> *The first step toward long-term change is being aware of your own bullshit and denial!*—Dr. Barry Weichman

Men and emotions are no longer oil and water, which don't mix—our relationships can be psychologically balanced. We need to increasingly mix, match, and understand that our quality of life is a nonstop process. I end this chapter with two stories about men and the processes of developing their emotional intelligence, psychological balance, and mental health.

TWO STORIES OF MALE VULNERABILITY

Jax's Story of Complete Transparency

Jax, age thirty-eight, was raised by two lesbian mothers in an affluent community on the East Coast. Jax never met his father, who was a sperm donor. He had very little exposure to men and masculinity growing up. Jax decided around age ten that he was going to learn how to be a "man." He started playing football and continued playing through college, where he majored in business and dated only "hot" women. Yet he always felt a deep uneasiness about his parents and "weird" family background, and he always felt "different."

Jax, gifted athletically, found sports to be both a blessing and a curse. Jax didn't want anyone to know that his parents were two mothers. He told his friends growing up that his dad had died before he was born. The big secret came out in middle school, and he was bullied until his junior year of high school for having gay parents. Jax confronted the three bullies who had spray-painted his school locker florescent, hot pink. He challenged the bullies and his entire football team for being homophobic—no one argued the point. After this emotional moment for Jax, no one ever challenged him again. Jax told the leader of the bullies that he would not allow it anymore.

Jax, who was not a bodybuilder, was not afraid of directly confronting the issue or his bullies.

The psychological courage to stand up to the bullies—his male peer group—and confront the rumors forever changed his life. He chose to be vulnerable and honest, not aggressive or defensive about his two mothers. The irony is that several of his teammates had similar family dynamics. The mantra of honesty, vulnerability, and being kind has guided Jax throughout his life. Jax didn't avoid the difficult issues of his life, such as his family background, which has been rewarding though scary. Jax felt different because his family was not traditional, but at the same time he knew he was (and is) loved and understood.

After college, Jax started his own consulting business, married in his mid-twenties, and has two adolescent boys. Jax has debunked the stereotype that a boy without a father couldn't be a loving, caring, strong adult man. Having two lesbian mothers gave Jax the template for psychologically processing difficult emotions and awkward situations to understand his own feelings.

Josh's Story of Confronting His Father

Josh, age twenty-two, was a recent college graduate living with a few roommates and eating canned tuna for dinner. Josh got a remote medical insurance billing job to start supporting himself. The job was nothing Josh had ever considered or wanted, but being desperate and "broke," the job was a gift. His father, Peter, told Josh that he was a "loser" and an embarrassment to him and the family. The conversations with Peter became increasingly volatile and demeaning. Peter's only advice for solving Josh's problems was for Josh to go to law school and follow Peter's footsteps. Josh never considered being a lawyer a viable plan.

After several weeks of escalating tension, Josh finally confronted Peter about his inability to see Josh as his own person, not an extension of Peter. The call ended abruptly. They stopped talking for a few weeks. Early on a Sunday morning, Josh received an email from Peter informing him that Peter was cutting him off from all financial support. Peter also demanded to be repaid for all four years of Josh's college tuition. Josh, a recent college graduate with no savings, panicked.

Growing up, Josh always feared that if he disagreed with his father, he would cut him off emotionally and financially. Josh never expressed his true emotions or allowed himself to be vulnerable with his father because of Josh's fear about what his father would do if Peter didn't like what was said or discussed.

After the threatening email, Josh finally told his father, who was a senior partner in a worldwide law firm, that he was never going to be a lawyer. Josh abandoned his love of art, graphic design, and anything creative in high school to please his father and in the hopes of being loved. Josh realized that he was living his life for his father's approval and love, while becoming increasingly more depressed and miserable. Josh was scared to share his thoughts and feelings with anyone for fear of being rejected. Dating and friendships were scary for Josh, because he shared only what he thought the other person wanted to hear.

That fateful Sunday morning was the rejection and abandonment Josh always feared from his father. As painful, devastating, and terrorizing as it was, Josh didn't die. He had lived with the belief that if his father rejected him, his life would be ruined. Josh slowly began to realize in the following weeks and months that this blowup was perhaps the start of a new chapter. Josh's courageous decision to be direct and honest with himself first and then with Peter was the turning point in his life. Psychological honesty, emotional stability, a better understanding of himself, and decreasing depressive episodes were all immediate benefits of Josh's commitment to his masculine journey.

Personal Question

What scares you and prevents you from disclosing your deepest concerns, fears, losses, and hopes to a close friend? (Jax and Josh did it, and they didn't die nor will you.)

CHAPTER SIX

MEN AND SHAME

Emotional Cancer, the Silent Killer

Failure is success in progress.—Albert Einstein

The measure of intelligence is the ability to change.—Albert Einstein

M en and the topic of shame are gaining more mainstream attention and focus. The quotes above are reminders that change is possible in spite of the insidious nature of shame: feeling defective, damaged, fraudulent, and unlovable. Shame is a universal experience and is universally misunderstood. Shame isn't guilt! Guilt is action that can be corrected. Shame is a negative belief or emotion that is constant regardless of outside actions to offset it. Shame lives and thrives within a man's psychological operating belief system, which influences his emotional response. The skewed perception of people and your daily interactions creates negative misinterpretation of one's own and others' feelings, moods, and other people's behaviors. Shame is a psychological condition that requires treatment, just as depression, anxiety, trauma, and eating and personality disorders.

> *Denial, anger, violence, and amnesia are symptoms of avoiding the awful shame-based emotions of feeling like damaged goods, an imposter and unlovable.*

Shame functions as a poisonous element that distorts and psychologically cripples men, inside and out. Shame is viewed as a secondary cause, not a primary factor for mental illness or maladapted antisocial behaviors. Men (me included) tend to dismiss the fact that shame is a major driving force in the development of toxic, abusive narcissistic masculinity—women know this and want the pattern to stop. The formal definition of shame is provided later; let's first describe some of its more common manifestations in men.

The unimaginable heart-wrenching stories of men walking into shopping malls, college campuses, an ex-wife's home, a workplace, and family parties with assault rifles are beyond comprehension. Absolutely no argument can be made that male violence isn't a mental health crisis driving these men toward deadly outcomes. Make no mistake: shame is a part of men's mental health crisis.

Shame is disguised as a bad feeling, but it is psychological cancer eating away at the fabric of your soul.

One piece of this complex puzzle of mental illness and mental health is the role that shame plays in men's psychology. The short answer is that shame is the "mud" covering up the gold brick inside a young man's heart and soul. Shame adversely affects the core personality growth of a man so that he is unable to properly view himself or his relationships. The degree of shame varies from person to person, but it is present until otherwise addressed. The understanding and natural development of a man's masculinity, career, financial growth, love relationships, and physical appearance is often viewed in the absence of shame. The self-loathing overlay of dreaded fear is one of the ways shame aborts healthy masculinity growth.

A man who gets out of his car with a baseball bat and smashes another driver's windshield during a moment of insanity is a classic example of untreated shame via rageful outburst. The expressions of "craziness" are many; the underlying feelings buried beneath these acts of aggressive, self-defeating choices and rage is shame. The problem or circumstances are not anger management problems.

All anger management issues and self-defeating behaviors are male aggressive traits disguised as untreated shame. Behavioral management coping skills for anger and domestic violence are effective and very useful in treating this psychological disease. The common denominator in all of these counterproductive actions and skewed psychological beliefs is shame, not depression or anxiety.

Shame/anger and emotional vulnerability are incompatible.

Unconscious automatic overreaction (i.e., screaming at the waiter, punching your teenage son) are generated from feelings of powerlessness, internal unease, and negative mood swings, which are problematic and dangerous. A skewed paranoid shaming perspective of your life leads to violent reactions, inappropriate social behaviors, abusive relationships, and ultimately deadly behaviors (suicide and murder). If a man's psychological core belief is "I am damaged goods," this negative self-image will increasingly distort, misdirect, and kill him inside and out literally and figuratively. This might sound extreme, but it isn't. *Shame is a serious mental health problem for men.* Men struggling with a shame-driven lifestyle are the equivalent of a nuclear handgun that only becomes increasingly more dangerous, toxic, and self-destructive over the years. Shame is not a minor wound or a temporary illness, nor is cancer. These emotional and physical illnesses are deadly and keep growing until there is an intervention. No intervention? No change, and no healing.

According to the American Medical Association, there are more than one hundred different types of cancer. These different types of cancer have a wide range of symptoms, which physically manifest in multiple ways. Shame, which is a psychological illness, also manifests in many different forms, reactions, beliefs, emotions, choices, and expressions. Shame commonly disguises itself in various forms of abuse, narcissism, depression, anxiety, unformed masculinity, and verbal outbursts. These all-too-common "guy" behaviors typically are dismissed as "men being men," Unfortunately, these self-defeating actions, negative emotional reactions, and troubled professional and personal relationships have their roots and foundation in a shame-driven personality.

DEFINITION OF SHAME—WHAT IS IT?

The typical behaviors of shame, their emotional blocks, and the despair that men experience are problematic and scary. The first hurdle is the lack of clarity and misunderstanding surrounding the underlying pathology of shame. Men from age sixteen to seventy-eight tell me week after week that they don't understand why they behave, think, or feel the way they do. In order to clear the mud and debris of shame off our life path, let's begin with the working definition of shame. For our purposes, shame is defined as:

> a primary emotional wound, not a secondary belief, based on a particular action; a paralyzing emotional, mental, psychological state of mind that distorts a man's view of himself and his daily life with others, preventing him from developing a healthy sense of self; impairing the man from developing trusting, secure, safe, loving relationships that are based on mutual respect and understanding; having a chronic emotional state of fear of being discovered as a phony, a fraud, and an imposter; prone to anger outbursts, embarrassment, or avoidant behaviors when feeling shame; the constant belief that you are "damaged goods."

(See my book *The Shame Factor: Heal Your Deepest Fears and Set Yourself Free* for more details on the subject.)

Shame question 1: What part of the shame definition can you relate to yourself?

Maybe you feel that you don't have any emotional or psychological shame issues or hinderances? We are going to take a self-rated test of our own psychological shame response cycle. The scale is an overview of some of the common reactions and the different appearances that our shame might take when overlaid with distortion, anger, and resentment. Shame is experienced in degrees of severity ranging from none, mild, average, moderate, moderate plus, severe, and extreme.

The problem with shame is the insidious nature and the difficultly of separating it from our "normal" psychological and emotional functioning. After many years of avoiding and experiencing self-doubt and embarrassment about having emotional needs, we become a prisoner of our deepest fears and unspoken insecurities—this is the crisis now facing men. Talking about our shame is a scary prospect and a powerful step toward creating a stable psychological foundation, which impacts every area and minute of our lives. Shame can't survive or control your life when exposed by its victim—you!

Shame question 2: How does shame impact or influence your life and your mental and physical health choices?

Before taking our self-evaluated shame test, let's further discuss how shame aborts personal vulnerability, transparency, and intimacy by first building a wall around your inner boy. Shame functions and exists in every type of relationship: personal, professional, family past and present, colleagues, casual and close friendships, and our relationship with ourselves. Shame can appear as "people pleasing," "approval seeking," extremely guarded, aloof, overly friendly, without personal boundaries, self-harming, and addictions of all kinds. The psychology of addiction is avoiding the uncomfortable, intolerable, and awful reactions to feeling "bad," hence we create ways to numb ourselves. These self-imposed behaviors have their genesis in our formative years of childhood and adolescence.

> *Chaotic childhood creates the internal voice: "I am bad, no one loves me, and I am a failure," which is the onset of developing feelings of shame and inadequacy.*

The suppression, denial, and forgetfulness of unresolved pain, instability, and childhood abuse can be found in every type of addictive behavior. For example, chronic marijuana use, recreational cocaine use, hallucinogenic drugs, chronic gaming, gambling, online shopping, chronic pornography use, social media addiction, scrolling, injurious behaviors (i.e., cutting yourself, bulimia), and physical altercations. *These behaviors and many more like them are purposeful!* All behaviors serve a purpose—negative or positive. The question is, what's the purpose of your conscious and unconscious behaviors? I don't want us to get lost in the weeds or caught up in the minutia of useless details that avoid the issue at hand: your shame and your emotional transformation.

The following examples are a few cleverly disguised shame-based behaviors that may seem harmless and that you may have been told were unchangeable or a personality trait.

- Extreme panic/fear response to criticism
- Extreme mood swings—joy, impending doom, or feeling defective
- Raging outbursts—overreacting to minor events
- Road rage—driving aggressively and feeling violated/offended by other drivers
- Overspending—wanting or needing to have the newest things
- Conflict avoidance—fearful of upsetting, disappointing, or letting others down
- Inability to express contrary opinions in your romantic relationships—prone to seeking the approval of others regardless of your own feelings
- Needing to make everyone happy in order for your world to feel safe
- Overworking to avoid your personal life—no personal boundaries
- Your family blames you for their problems and issues, triggering your rage, creating an endless cycle of self-loathing and self-doubt about yourself
- Regular drug or alcohol use to "numb" yourself, with no regard for the dire consequences of your choices
- Compulsive overthinking about problematic future scenarios or impending doom

Circle at least three of the behavioral descriptions above that describe you or that are examples of things that you do. These behaviors might not seem problematic or like emotional blocks to your mental and psychological health. Don't be fooled or drink the shame Kool-Aid of denial, avoidance, and fear.

It's imperative to remember that shame and change aren't friends; they resist each other. Our inner voice of self-doubt and insecurity will scream at us to never expose them or confront the lie fueling them. Courage is asking yourself the tough questions about your feelings of shame and its role in your life.

Shame question 3: Why do you do certain things that aren't in your best interest?

Shame question 4: How do you feel about these actions and habits (good, numb, sad, etc.)?

Shame question 5: When and how did these certain behaviors and habits begin?

One of the biggest questions in the field of human behavior, psychology, and social science is why do we do the things we do? One answer is that the primary purpose underlying addictive behaviors and addictions is to suppress, avoid, deny, and dismiss the paralyzing feelings of shame. Think about this for a minute: our internal survival instinct is so sophisticated that we create barriers, which we might not even be consciously aware of, to protect our psychological self.

> **All our behaviors, choices, and reactions serve a purpose. Nothing you do is without a purpose!**

Our list of behavioral reactions to shame are typically viewed as something other than unspoken beliefs about feeling inferior, flawed, or bad. You can't outrun, outwork, or outthink your uncomfortable sense of feeling damaged, fragmented, or disposable. These types of unspoken psychological beliefs began in our childhood and early parent-child relationship. The disappointments, emotional neglect, traumas, and physical neglect are now buried deep within our man cave of silence. We create automatic, reflexive addictive behaviors for *never* re-experiencing these paralyzing waves of our own brand of shame—this includes me and anyone else who has stared down their reasons for feeling, believing, and experiencing their own emotional terror-shame.

The idea of being emotionally vulnerable, transparent, and psychologically insightful is a scary proposition, one that many men avoid with tremendous effort and pain. Many men choose to be isolated rather than to ever risk the potential of feeling powerless or shamed in a relationship. Collectively these choices and behaviors create a fractured, hollow masculinity within. It's impossible to feel psychologically stable and emotionally grounded when you have a nagging fear that eventually everyone will discover that you are really an imposter pretending to be a high-functioning loving adult man. You can't let anyone get too close for fear they will discover your secret: of not being "enough." Noah's story below is a prime example of what happens when you avoid, deny, and pretend that you have no issues to resolve.

Before we go any further, I want you to know firsthand that male shame-driven actions are amendable to treatment. Nothing in your life—not your mental health or your relationship world—is beyond healing and transformation. I am going to give you the tools, information, and courage to wash off the mud of shame covering up your best self—your inner gold brick! Your heart and soul are waiting for your transformation. The following sections of the book are ongoing practical solutions for this intangible sick feeling and for building your masculinity from within. We first uncover your shame cycle and what it looks and feels like for you.

A CAUTIONARY TALE—NOAH'S ANGER ISSUES WITH WOMEN

Please note that the following story contains sensitive sexual material.

Noah's story is a compelling illustration of unresolved childhood trauma with no expiration date. The negative impact of shame and its residual distortion of one's relationships and self-image are viewed through a cracked psychological lens. The unmentionable, unhealed, and unexamined trauma layered with shame creates a constant sense of feeling overwhelmed, damaged, and anxious. From about age seven, Noah was taught how to give his babysitter—a female cousin ten years older than him—back rubs while straddling her back. Noah recalls at the time he thought it was "weird" that she wanted him to do it on her bare back. He didn't want to make her mad, so he learned how to do the back rubs. The back rubs continued until he was approximately fourteen years old, at which time Noah was becoming sexually aroused while doing them. His cousin made moaning sounds when he rubbed her back, and finally he couldn't do it any longer. Noah had told his parents about this situation many times before, and they assured him that it wasn't a problem. Noah started drinking after school in eighth grade to avoid his cousin.

When Noah refused to give any more back rubs to his now-adult cousin, his mother began to pressure him to give her back rubs instead. Noah's mother told him that she was jealous that he wouldn't give her the same type of attention. Noah remembers becoming sexually aroused for the first time at around eight years old with his cousin. Finally, as a teenager, the situation became too "freaky and sick" according to Noah, and he refused to cooperate anymore.

Noah never gave his mother a back rub nor his cousin after coming home drunk after school one day and passing out in the family room. Noah's father ignored his pleas to send him away to boarding school so that he could avoid his cousin and mother. The pressure he felt from his mother to give her a back rub was present until he left for college at eighteen years old.

Fast forward to age forty-two: Noah stopped drinking several years earlier after twenty years of "slowly" killing himself with bimonthly ten-day drinking binges. Noah went to college and dated only high-drama women who also were heavy drinkers. The cycle of drinking and the pattern of volatile relationships continued into his marriage. Noah's wife stopped drinking when she got pregnant with their five-year-old daughter. After six years of marriage, she left him (the reason for our therapy sessions) because of his anger outbursts and raging verbal abuse about how "awful" women treat him.

In the coming months, Noah and I met several times a week to address the embarrassment and humiliation he felt concerning his sexual trauma. Whenever Noah became overwhelmed during our sessions with emotions (i.e., anger, sadness, fear, and disappointment), his default response was, "Dr. P., get serious. Guys aren't victims of sexual abuse. They get over it, and it is not a problem." In order to further discount, dismiss, and avoid his feelings, Noah would say in a sarcastic, cynical tone of voice, "Who gets to give a back rub to his sexy hot-looking cousin and doesn't enjoy it? I am messed up because now I would love it."

Every time he would digress into a shaming self-loathing moment, I remind Noah that he is now a fortysomething adult man, a law firm partner, and financially independent, not a scared, confused eight-year-old boy whose story no one believes. The young boy inside of Noah had no idea of why he felt the things that he experienced until adulthood. Noah told me after a few sessions that his cousin died several years ago from cancer. He didn't understand why he felt sad and a sense of loss when he learned about her death rather than celebrating it.

Cancer is physical rebellion against the body. Shame is psychological rebellion against the self.

YOUR SHAME SCALE

The discussion of toxic masculinity versus healthy masculinity, men's mental health issues, and the crisis of being a man can be addressed head-on with a deeper understanding of how shame affects our life. Mass shooters (99.999 percent are men), fathers who murder their families, and men who sexually assault women—not to overstate the obvious—are all struggling with serious mental health issues. Mixed into this cocktail of mental illness is the nuclear ingredient of shame. Make no mistake: shame is as dangerous as any other mental health challenge and is given the least amount of attention.

The reasons for this are many, but for our purposes let's agree that discussing shame is as uncomfortable a topic a man will ever discuss (again, put me on that list).

Our shame has roots in our deepest, darkest, and most revealing aspects of ourselves. Shame is the ugly part of ourselves that we are afraid to look at or even acknowledge. The ugliness is the illusion of avoidance and secrecy. Who wants to talk about their sexually abusive neighbor growing up or the football coach who touched your body?

No one. Until the psychological tumor has become too big, too painful, and too damaging to ignore. Noah is a prime example of men who would rather skip over embarrassing childhood events and discuss sports, work, and golf. We discussed the need for men to be more emotionally engaging, vulnerable, and insightful for themselves and others. The only way this is going to happen is to clear the debris off our life path. This implies that we begin clearing off the mudslide of shame choking our core self. When the elements, variables, and emotions of shame are understood, exposed, and addressed, new opportunities abound.

Shame blocks us from us—we are unable to experience peace of mind and contentment.

Until our shame is addressed, it will be our own personal terrorist rebelling against the development our best self, personal potential, and secure relationships. Shame's purposeful blockade of our psychological stability, mental health, and quality of life can be compared to a cancerous tumor—the tumor has to go! We know that untreated, undiagnosed tumors continue to grow, damage, impair, and ultimately take the life of their victims.

The throbbing headache, back pain, prostate problems, lumps under our arms, and stomach ulcers are early warning signs that something in our body isn't right. Men, we are notorious for ignoring these physical, flashing-red warning signs, as we discussed earlier in this book. The same analogies hold true for our emotional cancer growths, which seem harmless until we are terminated from our job for anger-management problems, or arrested for domestic violence, or consider suicide, or buy a gun for revenge against an ex-romantic partner.

It's apparent that shame is a dangerous psychological variable that needs to be resolved, or at least reduced, in its potency and control of your life. The following scale itemizes graduating degrees of shameful emotions, actions, and beliefs. It should be noted that your experience of shameful emotions, actions, and reactions can be episodic and situationally dependent, not a daily occurrence.

Your Shame Scale, 0–10

0—You have no emotional reaction to critical feedback, authority, or change of plans and no sense of self-loathing or negative self-talk. You accept difficult situations, uncomfortable discussions, and differences of opinion. You feel emotionally neutral about the people who disagree with you. You enjoy being emotionally connected and vulnerable with others.

1—You understand in your mind the concept of shame in regard to feeling bad about the past. You don't allow your shame to control money matters, relationships, arguments, or how you express your frustrations. People aren't scared of you when you are upset or angry. You enjoy different types of people and social situations.

2—You occasionally feel bad about yourself; maybe you fear that you are an imposter, fooling everyone in your life about your stability and maturity. Your feelings of self-doubt don't last very long and are offset by positive psychological beliefs and positive actions for yourself and others. You enjoy your life and present-day circumstances. You have a sense of gratitude, and it stops your cycle of shameful feelings.

3—You are aware that certain people, events, or family situations trigger aggressive reactions followed by a wave of shameful emotions. You deny that these situations have any underlying or unresolved issues from your past. You feel empowered to openly hate and resent your ex-partner and jokingly threaten them. You quickly forget the situation and the awful emotions that you felt. You are generally very positive until a wave of shame hits you.

4—You rarely reveal personal information about yourself or voice unpopular opinions. You are a very private person with a "no-problem" public persona and are everyone's friend. You secretly fear being embarrassed and exposed as a fraud (distorted personal self-image). You avoid close relationships including romantic and keep everyone at arm's length to avoid seeing inside of you. You fear that you are "damaged goods" beyond repair and unlovable.

5—You have unexplainable bouts of rage at others; you hate yourself and are physically violent. You fear being seen as a weak, pathic, or bad person. You are constantly worried about any relationship issue, minor or major, for fear of being rejected. Your emotional overreaction to disappointment is disproportional to the event or situation. You have uncontrollable negative verbal rants toward yourself when people in your life are unhappy with you. You don't believe anyone truly loves or cares for you.

6—You feel angry, upset, and irritable with everything and everyone more days than not. You have waves of shame about what people think of you. You try to hide your insecurities and self-doubt with a false image of perfection to the world and to your partner, family, and close friends. You have secrets and a secret life. You avoid issues until you are screaming or yelling. Avoidance and ignoring your feelings is normal for you. You don't allow anyone to truly know you.

7—You are unable to control your emotions when someone blames or accuses you or questions your actions. You immediately feel shame then respond aggressively and defensively when you feel that you are being judged or wrongly evaluated. You panic emotionally whenever you feel exposed or at fault for something. You try to maintain a perfect image to the world until your rage, resentment, and despair overwhelms you. People are scared of your anger, hostile mannerisms, and aggressive verbal attacks. You "go off" when you feel wronged or neglected. Your partner believes you have anger issues or untreated bipolar disorder (extreme mood swings).

8—You are prone to making threats or becoming involved in physical altercations when you are upset. You use excessive force via guns, bats, and weapons to intimate people. You choose to have no emotional insight into your behaviors and reactions. You know you struggle with anger, rage, and violent mood swings. You have physically beaten, hurt, or hospitalized someone in a fit of rage. You are very sensitive to people's opinions of you and react violently when you feel "disrespected." A restraining order has been filed against you by a former partner. You have been arrested. You have a history of violence in the workplace or of domestic violence; You crave approval but will not allow anyone to know that. You drink or use drugs on a regular basis to offset your awful feelings. You carry a gun for protection in non-dangerous situations.

9—Your life is controlled by your unhealed shame. Your relationships to yourself and others are shaped and controlled by anger, resentment, violence. You feel ripped off by life. You hate your family, parents, former employers, and anyone else who has wronged you. You are unable to discuss differences of opinion without reacting defensively, aggressively, and, many times, without physical fighting. You have no tolerance for people who seem weak or frail.

You have been a victim of abuse as a child. You don't believe you can be helped other than by avoiding living near certain people: Your partner is scared of you. You believe your partner is unfaithful and you must control their actions. You don't express or understand your emotions. You do self-destructive things to yourself via drugs, reckless behavior, and poor health. You feel very bad, hate yourself, and cover it up with aggressive, tough-guy actions.

10—You hate yourself. Your life is a series of violent encounters and shame-based actions that are impulsive, dangerous, and possibly deadly. You consider suicide and murder as options for solving your problems. You have attempted suicide before. You have been physically abused and have been physically abusive as adult. Your friends share and support your aggressive beliefs, antisocial behaviors, and violence. Your relationships are based on partying, violence, and crime. You have negative emotions that you suppress with rage, anger, and deadly force. You have been arrested for violent crimes. You are unable to keep a legal job because of your issues with authority, theft, and fraud. You blame others for your hard life and current problems. You misrepresent yourself to others in order to gain advantage over them. You believe that your life will end soon. You don't allow anyone to be close to you. Your relationships are based on power, control, and force.

SUMMARY

Our masculine shame scale is a window into the dangers of untreated shame. Unfortunately, untreated cancer and untreated shame both result in dire outcomes for the sufferers. Please don't be offended by or dismissive of these ten windows into the mind of a shame-driven man. It's a serious psychological condition that requires action, understanding, and self-acceptance.

In our vignette, Noah was embarrassed and confused about being a victim of sexual exploitation. The emotional denial caused by his internal shame ultimately blew up his life. Noah's story dispels the myth that "real men" can't be victims of sexual abuse and rape. Experts in the field of sexual abuse and trauma know that men underreport incidents of sexual abuse. Men's reluctance and resistance to acknowledging any type of abuse or trauma are the biggest roadblocks to healing.

From the outside looking in, Noah had it all: money, prestige, and power. Yet what he really was living with was despair, embarrassment, self-loathing, rage, and a love-hate relationship with women. None of these psychological variables lends themselves to emotional clarity or mental stability, Noah feeling desperate to save himself, his marriage, and family, started with addressing his traumatic shame-inducing childhood.

We know shame left untreated can destroy a man's life literally and figuratively. You are the only person who can stop the cycle of shame from passing on through you to your family. You cannot function mentally, psychologically, and emotionally with shame controlling you.

In chapter 7, I address how to begin to recognize, heal, and stop the violent outcome of unrecognized, untreated shame, the seven common triggers of shame, and the deadly expression of shame for men.

CHAPTER SEVEN

HEALING THE CYCLE OF MALE VIOLENCE

Stopping the Emasculation Process

You will continue to suffer if you have an emotional reaction to everything that is said to you. True power is sitting back and observing everything with logic.—Bruce Lee

One of the most important abusive relationships we need to transform is the one that we have with ourselves.—Xavier Dagba

EMOTIONAL IQ FACTS FOR MEN

- Emotional vulnerability is the doorway to greater insights and mental health fitness.
- Unresolved "stuff" continues to fester and disrupt your emotional life until you confront it.
- Shame is your own critical, internal "terrorist."
- Psychological and emotional healing starts from within then manifests in your in actions, behaviors, and choices.
- Fear breeds a smaller and smaller life experience for you.
- Anxiety lies to you—every disappointment isn't urgent or catastrophic.
- Emotional bonding, peace of mind, and secure personal and professional friendships are choices.
- Men are as emotionally capable and have the same fundamental emotional needs as women.
- Expressing your feelings is curative and allows for your transformation.
- Men need emotional connections and meaningful discussions with other men.
- Greed and selfishness breed emotional instability and self-deception.
- Male violence is a reaction to and symptom of unresolved shame.

- Toxic masculinity is the expression of the controlling selfish nature of shame-based masculinity.
- Insight about yourself and understanding others is psychological maturity.
- Emotional abuse (victim-perpetrator) is a repetitive pattern until it's resolved.
- Violence can't exist without shame.

These psychological facts are reminders of the powerful emotional capacity that men have within their lives. Men who wisely choose to use their words rather than resort to aggressiveness during a confrontation aren't passive or powerless. Instead, this is an example of genuine positive masculine influence, of self-control and respect for others during a heated encounter. Accessing, developing, and using only a small portion of your psychological-emotional potential is a tremendous loss to you and your world of influence. We need to have all four quadrants of our life fully functional to maximize our potential and fulfill our life path—physically, emotionally, relationally, and personally. These aspects are connected together in our masculine journey.

We unknowingly limit the overall quality of our lives by dismissing the wealth of potential that psychological stability can give us. Avoiding the intrinsic value of your emotional intelligence is like dying of thirst while swimming in a freshwater lake! Sounds odd but think about it. Let's consider some emotional roadblocks, denial, traumatic issues, and the untapped resources within you in this chapter.

> *Women want their men (i.e., partner, sons, brothers, father) to be emotionally intelligent, not the alternative!*

It's important for us to remember that the women—partners, daughters, mothers, and sisters—in our lives want their men to be masculine, self-accepting, and courageous, with a purpose in life. Women in couples therapy ask me all time why their husband/partner avoids their loving emotional invitations to talk, hold each other, and to share. How is this possible? Who would choose suffering and isolation, rather than tapping into emotional peace of mind?

Women want their man, sons, brothers, cousins, and guy friends to step into their potential. Men need to stop emasculating themselves in order to be seen as "safe" while avoiding their own personal needs. Allowing society to render men psychologically neutered promotes two extremes of male emotional intelligence: passive-helpless and aggressive-abusive! Emotional balance, personal growth, and understanding of others is aborted when we emasculate ourselves, hoping to be viewed as "nonthreatening" by the important women in our life.

The opportunity to be the psychological "rock" for the family, for your wife/partner, and most importantly for yourself doesn't have to be wasted; it's absolutely possible. It's never too late to start again on the highway of your life, regardless of how long you have been living in the "weeds" of your confusion. The desire to be an emotionally balanced man reaps huge dividends in your life; for example, in romantic relationships in which you and your partner can be vulnerable and create a strong supportive union, rather than one partner (you) being secretly afraid to be seen, while the other is hoping for emotional vulnerability. We are genetically wired to be in relationships, which provides the foundation for us to thrive.

> *Our past emotional pain is our present emotional pain until we actively acknowledge it. Our past shame will continue to be our present-day life experience, until we resolve it!*

It makes no sense that men continue to buy into the predetermined emotional straitjackets placed on them by the older brotherhood to fit into a role, macho appearance, career, or social circle or team. Think about ignoring at least one-third of your mental-emotional potential and intuitive nature in order to not feel any discomfort. Hmm, no one buying a house would skip looking at the inside just because the front porch has a great bench on it.

Sounds ridiculous but it is how we have navigated our psychological-emotional life—looking the opposite direction while pretending, forgetting, and secretly hoping that the past stays in the past. The past is our present until we deliberately separate it with our full attention and effort. One of the biggest myths men tell themselves is that avoiding our trauma, childhood events, parent-child issues, health scares, deaths, losses, self-doubts, and the sense of feeling "not good enough" will allow us to feel safe and secure! If this was true, you would not be reading this book.

VIOLENCE IS THE BEHAVIORAL EXPRESSION OF TOXIC LEVELS OF SHAME

A serious, life-threatening side effect of emotional avoidance, denial, and rejecting your emotions, thoughts, and feelings is the development of violence. Negative thoughts, distorted emotional perceptions, and a bleak outlook on your life come together like a perfect storm of terror, personally, relationally, and socially.

Over time, unresolved shame becomes toxic—deadly—which leads to toxic masculinity.

Male violence isn't a new topic but one that is incredibly misunderstood and feared. The reasons are many and one of the biggest contributors to male violence is "toxic shame," which is often called "toxic masculinity." There is no toxicity within men without the cancerous presence of unresolved shame. Physically violent men, male abusers, and sexual predators all have one thing in common: shame! Shame becomes increasingly dangerous and deadly when ignored and dismissed as a minor emotional issue. Shame is about as harmless as blood in the water as a shark is fast approaching its victim—you.

WHAT'S GOOD SHAME AND GUILT?

In the last chapter, we discussed the definition of shame and its insidious nature. We introduced the shame self-reporting scale, which outlines the progressive destructive nature of shame. We expose the magnitude of shame as emotional cancer and its chronic disruptive punitive nature in our daily life.

Many people often ask, "What is good shame?" We know shame isn't guilt. For example, guilt is triggered by making an insulting comment to your brother in-law at a family dinner. The comment had an aggressive tone and your wife glared at you for doing it. The next day you feel bad because the comment wasn't necessary or kind. Your behavior wasn't in line with the kind of man and example you want to set for your family. Guilt comes from our core value system, our moral compass for how we function in the world. Guilt serves as a warning system when we are offtrack with ourselves and others. Feelings of guilt are related to external events, actions, behaviors, and particular choices we make. Guilt is emotion that is generated from events around you.

Good shame is an emotional state of mind that is generated by our moral guide, ethics, values, and personal beliefs. Good shame is part of our psychological operating system, which helps us to be honest with and to understand ourselves in the context of our intimate relationships: with business colleagues, present-day family, adult children, and friends. Good shame is a constant belief, a psychological perspective that breeds peace of mind, mental health balance, and an enduring sense of fulfillment. The other end of the shame continuum is toxic shame. The shame continuum has two bookends: good shame and toxic, destructive shame. I discussed in the last chapter the various degrees of shame, ranging from very little to extreme levels of rage, hatred, and violence toward oneself and others. The higher concentration levels of shame are progressively more dangerous to men and destroy their mental health.

The tough-guy masculine model of the past advocated for men to be aggressive, forceful, bold, and courageous. Shame disrupts men from developing and taking responsible actions, making empowering decisions, and being supportive, not a loose cannon scaring and worrying their families, partners, colleagues, and neighbors. We all know these types of men who are walking around with a loaded gun of rage pointed at themselves and the world.

Men's Mental Health Questions

- What is one recent example of "good shame"?
- What's a recent example of your shame/self-doubt impacting your relationships?
- What's one of your emotional rageful, angry situations?

TOXIC SHAME DEFINED

Our definition of shame from the last chapter applies here with an addendum, for clarification purposes, regarding the progressive nature of this emotional cancer—toxic shame:

> An emotional, psychological, and behavioral reaction that is consciously intended to cause harm to self or others. The experience and primary expression of toxic shame involves violence, dangerous actions toward loved ones, acquaintances, and in extreme cases innocent victims. The expression of enraged powerlessness can be personal, suicidal, or external with murderous intentions toward friends, family, coworkers, ex-partners, classmates, or certain ethic groups. The primary emotional motive is to rid oneself of awful feelings, whether employing nonfunctional means or positive solutions. The emotional distortion is a result of the man being psychologically dysregulated, emotionally unstable, having untreated mental health issues, and lacking insight into their condition and its negative impact personally and socially.

Men externally express their rageful actions, dangerous behaviors, and fateful choices toward others. When asked, can you name one female mass shooter in the United States? The answer is a resounding "no!" Men externalize their rage, and women internalize theirs. After the Uvalde school shooting at Robb Elementary School in Uvalde, Texas, on May 23, 2022, the second deadliest school shooting since Sandy Hook Elementary in Newtown, Connecticut, ten years earlier, the *Los Angeles Times* stated the following: "These young men often show signs of severe distress long before they open fire. But either no one intervenes, or the interventions that do occur aren't effective."[1] The research is consistent with the inability of men to monitor themselves when they are consumed and controlled by toxic levels of shame and destructive choices.

A Cautionary Tale—The Crazy Guy Next Door

Unfortunately, this short story is a common tale among men who know guys who are aggressive, threatening, and violent. The brotherhood of men knows these men and doesn't want to confront their "scary" behavior unless it's necessary. My client, Sammy, age twenty-eight, grew up in the Pacific Northwest. Sammy came to therapy after his fiancée threatened to break off their engagement unless he discussed his family tragedy.

The unspoken family event involving Sammy, his two younger brothers, and his mother took place when he was sixteen years old. Sammy told me the following story as if he was discussing the tax code—informational, not personal—with no emotion or energy in his voice:

> When I was sixteen, my father was shot in the chest while walking to our mailbox by our crazy neighbor. My dad and this guy never liked each other. My dad had confronted him many times for how he would yell and scream at his wife and children. The guy would threaten my dad and told him it wasn't his business or problem. My dad would tell the guy it's not right to threaten, physically abuse, and throw his children out of the house. My dad called the police many times, and legal charges were pending, and arrests had been made for domestic violence.
>
> I will never forget this fall Saturday afternoon; you could hear my neighbor yelling and hitting the walls in the house. My father called the police, who were coming to the house; in the meantime, my dad walked outside to get our mail. I remember seeing our neighbor run out of his house toward my dad with a shotgun. I screamed but it was too late, the guy shot my dad in the chest. He fell to the ground and immediately died. The police arrived and ordered the guy to put the gun down. He refused and shot at the police. They returned shots and he was immediately killed. Then it seemed like everything stopped. There was a silence, probably a few seconds; it felt like it was five minutes. It was a scary moment, and I just stared at my dad.

My mother ran outside to my father lying on the front lawn, screaming. I will never forget looking at my neighbor lying face down in their driveway, dead. I don't remember much after that day and the next few years. The family next door moved away shortly after the shooting. I really think the guy's wife was happy that her asshole husband was dead. Our family never went to therapy or counseling. It was like it never happened. My mom still lives in the same house, and my brothers don't seem phased by it either. Both of my brothers still live near my mom. I moved to Los Angeles for college and never moved back home.

Getting married has me starting to think about my dad's murder. My life has never been the same since that day. I miss my dad, but he did the right thing, standing up to our neighbor. My fiancée keeps telling me I have unresolved emotional trauma about my father's murder. She believes it's the reason I get enraged when I see men bullying others at work or socially. I finally believed her when my boss recently confronted me about a client issue, and I wanted to beat his face in. I have never questioned my aggressive reaction to abusive men. My fiancée tells me it's not normal and scares her. My younger brothers, when they come to visit me, have also gotten into several barfights with dudes who think they can push younger guys around.

I don't want my wife or children someday to ever experience my rageful outbursts or anyone else. Violence kills and I think I have anger management issues when I see a bully or a guy taking advantage of someone in a lesser position. I feel like I am fucked up because of my past and only a few of my friends know this story. I know it's stupid to think this [his father's murder] has gone away because I don't talk or think about it very often. I have told myself that but deep down know it wasn't true. When we first started dating, my fiancée almost broke up with me when I told her this story.

This story is heartbreaking for everyone involved. The residual despair, years later for all the adult children and the two widows, carried from this toxic masculine meltdown. In a wink of an eye, the lives of two families were forever changed with no good explanation for why.

Sammy was in my office because his fiancée didn't grow up with rageful men, and she wasn't going to accept it. Violence, screaming, and

Masculine fact: Death at the hands of men will never be considered plausible or compatible with healthy masculine values and balanced mental health!

fighting isn't part of her personal experience of men or in her family's history. These types of psychologically low-functioning men—hostile men—are unfamiliar and scary to her. She is a barometer for Sammy to see himself as separate from his father's death and the residual emotions associated with it. For good reason, Sammy readily admits that male violence can't be condoned or dismissed as "boys will be boys!"

THE TIMELESS NATURE OF TRAUMA AND SHAME

The purpose of your internal emotional military defense is to protect you from ever experiencing these intense feelings of loss, hopelessness, terror, and unimaginable sadness and disappointment. *Remember that your shame has a purpose, counterproductive as it is!* Your shameful beliefs and emotions keep your past hidden from conscious thought while simultaneously interrupting your present life. Odd, but the complexity of emotional intelligence growth requires the removal of shame from your psychological-emotional beliefs and your moment-to-moment feelings.

Your shame has a purpose in your life until it is resolved.

> You cannot achieve your way out of your childhood trauma.
> —Will Smith

Will Smith's quote is powerful, especially after his emotional meltdown on a live, internationally televised stage at the Academy Awards ceremony in March 2022. His outburst and impulsive behavior were life-changing for him, his wife, and his professional peer group. His actions during that ninety-second period of time have altered his career, family, finances, and personal and professional image. Will received a ten-year suspension from the Academy of Acting as a consequence of his lapse of judgment—we have all had them. No judgment about Will Smith, because we (men) know and understand the irrational thoughts we have and actions we take at times. Even if we don't acknowledge the connection between our past and present suffering, the irrational emotions that come from our unhealed traumas are real and undeniable. We all have said, thought, and done things similar to Will's moment of infamy, just not on a worldwide television stage.

Shame is trauma's best friend—sounds counterintuitive but it's true! The cumulation of emotional layers of fear upon fear—feeling defective, not good enough, and damaged—becomes psychological mud. The mud covers your traumatized soul (wounded boy) and hinders your potential as a man.

Men are quick to discount significant events that happen in the past or present day that women would never consider to be normal or remotely acceptable, such as Sammy's father's murder on his front lawn in front of his entire family and neighborhood. This is extreme, but concerning their trauma, men commonly respond dismissively: "It's no big deal, it's in the past, get over it!"

SIGNIFICANT LIFE-ALTERING EVENTS— TRAUMA OR JUST A BAD DAY?

The clinical definition of trauma according to the American Psychological Association is as follows: "Psychological trauma and mental trauma is an emotional response to a distressing event or series of events, such as accidents, rape, sexual abuse or natural disaster. Reactions such as shock and denial are typical."[2]

Dr. Esther Giller, president of the Sidran Institute wrote in her paper on trauma,

> Although I am writing about psychological trauma, it is important to keep in mind that stress reactions are clearly physiological as well (i.e., mind-body connection). Different experts in the field define psychological trauma in different ways. What I want to emphasize is that it is an individual, subjective experience that determines whether an event is or is not traumatic. Psychological trauma is a unique, individual experience of an event or enduring condition in which:
>
> • The individual's ability to integrate his/her emotional experience is overwhelming, or
> • The individual experiences (subjectively) a threat to life, bodily integrity, or sanity.[3]

An academic debate about the differences between a stressful event, abuse, and traumatic situation isn't relevant here. The issue isn't whether it is an isolated event, chronic drama, neglectful parenting in childhood, or adolescent drama. Maybe you don't consider it very serious. The issue is: What is the impact of your past traumas on your psychology currently?

The event might have been difficult to emotionally process, understand, or accept, as with Sammy's situation. The scary, abusive, enduring situations of instability, homelessness, divorce, and situations that were out of your control create emotional impressions of trauma on mind and emotions. Listed below are examples of trauma circumstances that are often discounted or devalued even though the psychological impact and suffering isn't diminished or reduced. Consider the possibility that the following events could be more than one-time events in your life.

- You lost your job, and you can't afford rent/mortgage.
- Your adult son is addicted to heroin and is homeless.
- Your wife has breast cancer.
- Your mother was a single parent who was resentful about your father.
- Your father was a single parent who spoke negatively about your mother and alienated you from her.
- Your best friend from high school died last week.
- You are going through a divorce and custody battle, and you are the bad guy!
- You are getting married, and the in-laws don't like you.
- You feel responsible for other people's happiness.
- You require major surgery.
- You owe more than $400,000 in school loans.
- You were sexually violated as young boy, and you never told anyone about it.
- You have erectile dysfunction with your wife/partner.
- Your adult children no longer talk to you.
- You are a domestic violence suspect or victim with a chaotic relationship/marriage.
- You have been in a life-altering accident or have a health condition and are unable to function at your previous levels of competency.
- Both of your parents have died.
- Your newborn child has medical issues requiring major surgeries.
- You are fifty pounds overweight and need back surgery.
- Your childhood was chaotic, and you are embarrassed about it.
- You were bullied throughout your school years.
- You witnessed a murder or are a victim of a violent crime.
- You have no money saved for your kid's college fund or retirement because of a bad business deal.
- You are more than forty years old and have never had a relationship last longer than three years.

Men's Mental Health Questions

- What is a stressor, person, or situation that drains your emotional energy?
- What in your past is something you feel very shameful about?
- When do allow yourself to relax?
- Does anyone know about traumatic events from your childhood, your adolescence, or your adult life?

The traumas listed above are a reminder of some commonly dismissed situations, past events, and present circumstances that are stressful. Your psychological state of mind is not feeling safe, is emotionally terrorizing, and feels traumatic. Fear causes us to overreact, lose our adult perspective of a situation that is objectively harmless but feels emotionally dangerous. A growing sense of doom, cumulation of catastrophic moments, and ongoing traumatic events occur throughout our lifetime, leaving us to resolve and manage them. Our emotional state of feeling unsafe is never fully understood or healed—the thoughts of the past and present day keep triggering our psychological-emotional reactions. Our emotional triggers have their origin in our traumatic darkroom of past events, which keep replaying in the present day.

Men will avoid their traumatic past experiences by overcompensating. No lasting relief or resolution comes from these diversions.

The male gag order of silence, which requires no emotional vulnerability and psychological insight, is compromised by the unresolved feelings within. Often, we become emotionally paralyzed with fear and shameful feelings of inadequacy, feeling defective and not good enough.

Those who feel emotionally powerless often react by sidestepping their emotional issues by overcompensating to appear invincible and powerful. These actions often translate into making enormous amounts of money, having sex with random women, prolific and dangerous drug use, buying exotic sportscars, houses, and other big-ticket items, and making impulsive business deals in order to feel powerful. All of these actions are reactions to the ugly feelings, thoughts, and emotions that our shame triggers.

These actions aren't wrong or psychologically unhealthy by themselves; it's the intention and purpose of these actions that are problematic. We know that external pleasures are never a long-term substitute for treating and accepting our emotional losses or disappointments. Dealing with our present-day issues helps us to see the emotional connections to the past that need our full attention, patience, and courage to resolve. A positive outcome of dealing with our "stuff" is a sense of feeling competent, which breeds self-confidence. Shame is powerless in the face of your sense of competency, courage, and self-confidence.

Men's Mental Health Questions

- Are there any events, situations, or childhood experiences that could be problematic in my life today?
- What's one of my self-doubts or imposter behaviors at work or with my friends?
- Is your unspoken secret from the past resolved or shoved into your man cave?

With thousands of years of social conditioning urging men to hunt or be hunted, to kill or be killed, a masculine perspective for physical violence has developed that excludes the capacity for emotional vulnerability. The guy who expresses any type of emotional vulnerability is considered weak, not fit for a man's job, not considered a leader. These ingrained beliefs have contributed to our current masculine crisis of how to be psychologically insightful, strong minded, and emotionally balanced. Excising 40 percent of our psychological abilities by experiencing only heated emotions rather than positive ones isn't a good idea for developing any degree of mental health balance, stability, and meaning in our lives.

> *Trauma comes back as reaction, not a memory.*—Bessel Van Der Kolk

Men need all "360 degrees" of their psychological capabilities to end the multigenerational cycle of emotional ignorance and emotional immaturity in the brotherhood. This is a wonderful time in human history for men to begin to fully access their innate psychological abilities and gifts and become valuable resources at home, at work, and for their family, friends, and their own lives.

HOW TRAUMA BECOMES ANGER

The quote above by Dr. Van Der Kolk is brilliant! Our overreactions, emotional outbursts, road rage, and mistrust of our partner are all trauma-anger responses and, as the quote above points out, not memories but visceral reactions. The loss of a loved one, being abused, and suffering neglect as a small boy are all significant events in your life. Sammy didn't consider his family situation traumatic or all that serious; rather, it was only something in his history. Until his girlfriend pointed out his exaggerated responses of rage to minor slights or the angry overaction to being cut off at the supermarket, Sammy wasn't aware of his untreated trauma—shame. The murder of his father wasn't at the front of Sam's mind, but the raw, emotional nerve of being a victim was! Whenever that nerve was touched, Sammy became a "monster" according to his girlfriend.

Men's Mental Health Questions

- Have any of your close friends, work colleagues, or family expressed concern about your "anger issues"?
- What's something that was significant to you during childhood or adolescence?
- When was the first time you felt embarrassed about yourself, your parents, or your siblings?

Our list of significant life events can be traumatic and disruptive to your life while growing up and to your life today. The old tough-guy masculinity lacks psychological courage—it's not in their wheelhouse of abilities. Tough-guy men reject men who express their feelings of sadness, fear, grief, and despair. Resisting our psychological health creates men lacking insight and lacking responsibility for the consequences of their impulsive actions. When we carry around years and years of emotional disappointment, loss, and trauma, we are unable to be vulnerable with others and incapable of being a positive partner, parent, or friend. We feel defective and are unconsciously controlled by our fear of being exposed.

A negative inner narrative of shame distorts the positive side of life. The inner lens of shame clouds our ability to see challenges with an open mind. Our clouded perceptions of our own value create psychological confusion about our relationships and the people we encounter. This distorted psychological view of our relationships evolves into our own crisis of not knowing how to live in the world peacefully. Our shame is our fear of life, living, and needing to protect ourselves from our demons and the people triggering them—this is how men become dangerous, violent, and deadly.

Repeated negative reactions by our wounded inner boys come out as rage, resentment, disappointment, feelings of inadequacy, paranoia, and greediness.

Men who feel powerless will revert to revenge as a tool to right the wrongs in their life. Seeking revenge against your ex-wife, parents, business partners, or anyone else is a deadly emotional-shaming cocktail. Unless there is a personal intervention, a dangerous wounded man is walking around like a ticking time bomb, hence toxic masculinity.

THE SEVEN CLASSIC TRIGGERS OF TRAUMA— OUR EMOTIONAL LEGACY

We have covered a lot of ground on accepting, removing, and creating a shame-free zone for your psychological-emotional growth. This is the pathway forward in developing a strong sense of yourself, empathy for others, your life plan, and belief in yourself and something bigger than yourself. Emotional intelligence is fluency in your own psychological language. Having insight into your emotions, feelings, and thoughts is priceless—it's one of your super-powers. You will begin to fully control how you want to navigate your personal life, career, health, family, and love life.

The seven emotional triggers reinforce our personal defense against feeling powerless, defective, small, damaged, or vulnerable! These feelings cause men to make bad decisions when they feel small.

1. Fear of embarrassment (emotional paralysis): Unable to be vulnerable with people; uncomfortable with any degree of openness, transparency, or honesty with others; hiding yourself so no one can see your imperfections; unspoken belief that you will be humiliated and hated if any knows your secrets, personality flaws, or chaotic background; extreme defensiveness and fear about any type of personal or professional exposure.
2. Feeling angry (disrespected and dismissed): Distorted view of yourself as a victim; inability to verbalize feelings of frustration without intense anger; unable to manage feedback; moody and emotionally volatile; prone to outbursts that are disproportional to the situation; personalizing others' actions as acts of aggression toward you; chronically defensive about your behavior.
3. Imposter syndrome (feeling like a fraud): Fear of being discovered as inadequate; chronic feelings of failure and fearful of losing your job; feeling useless at your job; fearful of being viewed as incompetent; unable to make mistakes; chronically fearful of others' motives or actions to discredit you; unable to take professional risks.

HEALING THE CYCLE OF MALE VIOLENCE **97**

4. Feeling isolated (fear of rejection): Self-selecting actions to keep emotional distance from people; a loner who is lonely, craving secure friendships but incapable of taking action to have them; socially uncomfortable; emotionally guarded with superficial relationships; unable to join groups for fear of being found out as defective.

5. Suspicious of authority (unable to trust people or their intentions): no close friends due to the belief that they will use you or take advantage of you; resentment issues with your parents; refusal to be in a subordinate place/ role for fear of abuse, exploitation, and feelings of emotional powerlessness; high unemployment history.

6. Fear of intimacy (belief that one is unlovable): Caretaker of your parents while growing up; unhealed abusive history; significant losses early in life; emotional neglect of self; self-harming habits; unstable emotional relationships; you blame yourself for others' actions or problems; fearful of your "secret" being discovered.

7. Fear of criticism (unable to tolerate disappointing others): Your choices have to be perfect; people-pleasing; placating and dependent on the approval of others; unable to value yourself or your actions; outwardly seeking love, acceptance, and approval; self-loathing and unresolved rage with a parent; hypersensitive to others' opinions of you; chronically uneasy when someone is upset or unhappy with you.

SUMMARY

The true profession of man is finding his way to himself.—Hermann Hesse

We have explored and uncovered the "mud" that keeps men from becoming who they desire to be and are capable of becoming. The doorway to becoming emotionally fluent with your own psychological process starts with clearing the debris off your highway in life. Emotional intelligence is achieved with emotional awareness, vulnerability, and resolving your challenges and traumas regardless of their severity. It should be noted that everyone has challenges; our narcissistic defense of appearing perfect can't survive the rigor of honesty, insight, and personal responsibility.

The cycles of anger fueled with shame are insidious and camouflaged as normal reactions. The poisonous nature of emotional anger-shame paralyzes is repeated trauma, which stalls out your journey to a fulfilling, healthy masculinity.

These seven cycles of emotional terrorism are the equivalent of gasoline on the fire of anger inside of you. Your particular triggers, beliefs, and visceral reactions are the ingredients of your struggles, fears, and personal hell-inducing roadblocks. Removing these barriers is the fast lane to withstanding, embracing, and experiencing the full range of your potential and ability to be loved and to love.

Men's Mental Health Questions

- What is one of my shame triggers that shuts me down?
- How does my anger impact my ability to have close male friends?
- What is something in my past that I need to talk about?
- Who are two men who know all—or most—of my secrets?
- How do I disconnect from myself (i.e., numbing out, social media, sex, drinking, sports, etc.)?
- What is one thing I am willing to do in the next twenty-four hours to emotionally connect with myself and a friend?

NOTES

1. Hayley Smith, Richard Winton, and Molly Hennessy-Fiske, "Texas School Shooting: 'State of Shock' as Uvalde Awaits Fate of Kids, Grieves, Prays," *Los Angeles Times*, May 24, 2022.

2. Kevin Rowell and Rebecca Thomley, "Recovering Emotionally from Disaster," APA, https://www.apa.org/topics/disasters-response/recovering, 2013.

3. Terry Hurley, "How Cognitive Processing Therapy for Trauma Helps Recovery," *Addiction*, November 16, 2017.

Part II

RELATIONSHIPS MATTER

You and Your Parents! Expanding Your Relationship IQ

Love is learning how to be vulnerable, not someone completing you!
—The Holistic Psychologist

*Sometimes, the things that break your heart end up
fixing your vision.*—Unknown

*A successful and healthy relationship does not mean the absence
of conflict, rather the ability and desire to work through it.*
—Dr. Jonathan Gottman, relationship expert

CHAPTER EIGHT

YOUR FATHER'S MASCULINITY

Why He Matters

I cannot think of any need in childhood as strong as the need for a father's protection.—Sigmund Freud, the father of psychotherapy

My father gave me the greatest gift anyone could give another person; he believed in me.—Jimmy Valvano, former Villanova University basketball coach

No relationship has had more of a lasting effect on me than my father. He died last year, and I regret spending the last thirty years proving him wrong, bad, and a loser. He wasn't any of those things; we just never expressed our love for each other.—Brett, age forty-three

FATHER-SON BACKGROUND INFORMATION—A TIMELESS BOND

Teenagers, twentysomethings, young adult men, and older men are unaware of the influence that their fathers have had in their lives. It seems obvious that young men become independent of their fathers; that developmental step happens around age fifteen. Boys leave home and get pushed out of the nest to find their way in the world, which seems like a natural end to the father/son chapter. Hmm, not so quick: this is when you begin to uncover the limitless influence of your father.

Career choices, your work ethic, male relationships, conflict resolutions, professional friendships, finances, sex, physical activities, health, and your relationship to women and children are your rights and responsibilities. We are going to call this all-encompassing influential relationship with your father the "father factor." Your father's influence is critical to gaining a full 360-degree understanding of your masculinity and all that it means to be a son, man, father, husband, brother, friend, and your own person.

Let's define *father factor* for our purposes as follows: The psychological foundation for your masculinity development, which functions in your career, your family, your mental health, your emotional intelligence, and your attachment style; the conscious and unconscious process of becoming a man; rules and guidelines to follow to become a man; your father's particular style of being a man forms your template for your masculinity.

NO CANCELING OUT YOUR FATHER FACTOR

Any discussion of fathers and sons is never going to be neutral or without some degree of sadness, regret, love, or acceptance. It's difficult, if not impossible, to fully understand your masculinity without acknowledging your father's influence. This can be a positive mixed with degrees of negativity and suffering in your life. Let me be abundantly clear: until you address head-on your father-son relationship, your capacity to maximize your potential professionally or personally will be limited. Having complete access to your masculine self and being the man you always wanted to be requires a visit to your father's symbolic home. The only way to solve any degree of resentment, anger, and sorrow and gain some resolution is to take a drive over to dad's house and begin a new dialogue between the two of you.

It should be noted that any man involved in your life when you were growing up who assumed the role of fathering you is a father factor. Biological fathers, stepfathers, and father figures are equally important for their critical roles in shaping your early years. Whomever you call "father" *is* your father. Remember that "stepparent" is a legal term, not a familial description.

GOING TO YOUR FATHER'S HOUSE

Before we go to dad's house, let's take a minute and address this death march toward the past (your past) with a myopic perspective of past, present, and the future. There is a current cultural movement to cancel, cut off, remove, annihilate, and erase people and things from our lives for past transgressions. Your relationship with your father is something you carry inside of you, and it cannot be removed or whitewashed with denial. Cancellation culture amounts to pouring gasoline on the barbeque and wondering why your dinner got ruined! It doesn't work!

You and father can be viewed objectively and compassionately and understood in the context of your past without malice or intent to abolish. I know there are chaotic family situations, fathers who are outliers from the brotherhood of parenting. We aren't discussing this small percentage of men, but rather the 95 percent of fathers and sons who want to have a better understanding of this unique relationship.

I encourage men of all ages to reconcile with your father within because he is a vital part of our life story.

Yup, we are going there. I suggest we drive over to his house, knock on the door, and plan on staying for a while. Let's not skip over your unspoken emotional needs (i.e., approval, feeling understood), which are buried somewhere along your road to success. Also let's not kick in his front door with blame, rage, or violence toward yourself or others. Please don't dismiss, minimize, or blame your father for the impact he has on your life today. Our entire discussion in this chapter about fatherhood is about taking personal responsibility for our lives with our father factor as the backdrop. Blame isn't part of our healing process or mental health balance.

Acceptance of your father is empowering. Blaming and resenting your father only prolongs the inevitable—forgiving your father!

Your father will always be part and parcel to your choice of whom to be or not to be. Either way, it's your choice as an adult man to resolve this all-important relationship regardless of the circumstances surrounding it. Let's do what is needed so you and the generations of men following you have positive male influences and leaders with balanced masculinity.

YOUR LIFE PLAN STARTS WITH YOUR FATHER

Casual conversations about our fathers can be superficial until our resentment starts to slip between the cracks of our wall of protection. When our resentment becomes active, disturbing our emotional well-being, that is a problem that can no longer be relegated to the basement of our life.

The insidious nature of resentment translates into feeling unlovable and not good enough, which gets stored inside our psychological thoughts and beliefs. Resentment and bitterness soon become a cement barrier blocking our natural development of growing up. Eventually our implicit or explicit issues with our father, such as physical/verbal abuse, divorce, finances, chronic criticism, unrealistic expectations, withholding love and support, evolve into a psychological paralysis within you. This process is universal across all cultures, races, education levels, economic situations, and types of fathers.

Our view and experience of men started with our fathers—never forget this fact. The first man that you loved was your father. Maybe the first man that you hated was your father. Either way, you are 50 percent your father, and it is worth your time and effort to glean as much information as possible from this relationship. I know that there are countless family situations with emotionally absent, neglectful, and critical fathers impacting their sons' early developmental years. Having the experience of a compassionate, mentoring, loving father or wanting to be a positive man/father impacting the world is based on you deciding how you feel as a son. Boys decide by age five or at the latest age eight whether they want to follow their father's emotional path or create their own.

The first man you loved was your father— whomever he is. Your model for being a man started with him, and understanding the magnitude of this relationship requires your full attention.

This decision includes seven basic emotional transactions between a father and son throughout their relationship. These seven relationship road markers are the bricks and mortar of your father-son connection. Every son carries a picture of himself that he takes into adulthood. This picture develops over the years with these building blocks that become the fabric of your masculinity, your relationships, your career path, and life choices. How the two men navigate these transactions is a barometer of how a boy's masculinity will evolve and how he feels about himself:

- Self-doubt versus feelings of competency
- Shame versus self-acceptance
- Fear of failure versus approval for living your life
- Emotional immaturity versus responsibility for your life
- Lack of focus/unpredictability versus balanced mental health
- Avoidance and anxiety versus a sense of independence/personal identity
- Anger/resentment versus emotional IQ

WHERE IT ALL BEGAN

Our early experiences with our fathers build our inner framework of being a man—masculinity. Every father-son relationship encounters seven emotional skills that impact who and what you are today—regardless of age. Your childhood, elementary school years, adolescence, and adulthood bear your father's influence and imprint. Your approach to every area of your life didn't happen in vacuum, but occurred in the context of you and your father's relationship. The short- and long-term emotional influence of your father can be an invaluable source of insight into your health habits, emotional disposition, body image, career path choices, sexuality preference, finances, romantic partner, and management/parenting style. It's time for us to turn our attention inward to the man you internalized as your role model—good or bad.

> *My mother raised me to always pick her over my father. My relationship with my dad had to go through my mother—this kept me away from my dad until they divorced when I was twenty-five years old. Then I met my father. He turned out to be a great guy.*—Stan, age thirty-six

We are all sons. Many times, we were raised to disregard our father for many reasons—let's not get lost in the weeds of family dynamics about your parents' marriage, divorce, and struggles. Stan's statement, unfortunately, is very common in distressed marriages where the children are used as emotional support for the parents. Professionally speaking, both parents are equally guilty of recruiting their children to compensate for the emotional gaps in their marriage or provide postdivorce support. Stepping aside from your parents' relationship with one another, let's focus on your independent relationship with your father.

Let's pause to think about your father apart from his relationship with your mom, sister, brother, and relatives or their opinions about him—just you and dad. Consider for a minute the untapped fund of knowledge your father-son bond holds for you. Most men, me included, waste many years skipping over this idea that our dad had anything valuable or positive to contribute to our lives. Regardless of your father's role in your life, there is information waiting for you to uncover.

FATHER-FACTOR QUESTIONS—YOU AND DAD

- What is your first memory of you and your father?
- When you think about your father, what are some of the emotions you feel?
- What does your father mean to you today?
- Did you feel or know that your father loved you?
- What character flaw do you and your father share?

- What trait do you respect in your father and yourself?
- What is something you would like your father to know?

OUR PRESENT-DAY MALE RELATIONSHIPS

Historically, our fathers and men are still largely defined by what they do outside the house. Men are the harshest critics of other men in terms of work, financial success, being good providers, leadership-social clout, their marriages, and fathering successful children. These measurements are brutal and don't represent the complete picture of being a loving adult man—just the appearance of an adult man—a huge gap in appearance versus substance.

What if your son struggles with addiction issues and drops out of high school and attends a drug rehabilitation program for two years? Then he attends trade school instead of your Ivy League university. Meanwhile your son is sober, alive, and developing a career for himself.

The stories, gossiping, and shaming are endless. Men judge other men for their own inadequacies. Men want other men to see only their strengths, not their vulnerabilities. Many times, in reaction to the ruthlessness of the brotherhood, we instinctively blame our fathers for our present-day struggles, even though they had no say in our present-day choices.

You watched everything your father did with a 24/7 mental video camera without knowing that you absorbed it.

Sons observe their father's work ethic, response to disappointments, choices and views about relationships, conflict resolution skills, and rule book for living. All these factors are written inside a son's heart and soul. Your father's nonverbal messages communicating how he viewed you are the baseline for your masculinity platform, which started when you were in your mother's womb. Men of all ages, me included, didn't know what we needed from our fathers growing up. Now as adult sons, we know what we didn't get from our fathers.

It's our responsibility to find the pathway to resolve this father wound in ourselves—in our masculine foundation. The path of least resistance is blaming and raging about our fathers. This choice is like pouring water on cement in the summer and wondering why it doesn't grow! Blaming and finger-pointing is very seductive. It gives the momentary illusion of resolve and relief from your emotional unease.

Regardless of their age, sons crave their father's approval, acceptance, and love!

The residual impact that our fathers pass down to us is a mix of positive elements—feelings of competency—simultaneously wrapped in painful emotional misunderstandings, self-doubt, and sadness. Fathers and sons often co-exist in an atmosphere of emotionally guarded silence and communicate with little or no heartfelt connections. The relationship is always acknowledged but its magnitude is difficult for both men to comprehend. What becomes painfully apparent for the son as he matures and enters his late teens and early twenties is the psychological, emotional, and mental need for his father's support and confidence in his ability to make a life for himself. I can't underscore enough this organic need that every son has for his father, father figure, or male mentor to believe in him.

Through daily actions and positive emotional interactions of feeling capable and understood, the son knows intuitively and verbally that he has his father's approval, acceptance, and love. A son who knows, feels, and experiences his father's invisible hand on his back are empowered, kind, compassionate leaders and mentors to other men.

> *The father-shaped wound in a man's life is a dangerous injury that has to be treated or it can become self-destructive, toxic, and deadly.*

Sons who grow up without these elements of validation, love, and understanding are missing critical pieces of their masculinity. The father-shaped wound often gets filled with rage, violence, and revenge to self and others. The resentment and rage for feeling unloved derails a young man's life. These boys who become adult men lack a sense of safety and a feeling of importance in the world. Unless they address their "father wound," these boys will continue to feel unloved, to feel like an imposter, and to become enraged. For example, many of these wounded boys grow up to become finance pirates, stealing from retirement funds to offset their emptiness, or violent abusers at home and in the workplace, resorting to dangerous means for feeling empowered.

These elements create a void in our souls and become feelings of self-doubt, lack of confidence, fear of living, depression, shame, and self-loathing. The psychological deficiencies that boys take into adulthood become the problems that they struggle to manage and heal throughout their life.

FATHER-FACTOR QUESTIONS—DEEP DIVE

- What did you want from your father growing up?
- What is something you desire from your father today (that isn't related to him living or dying)?

- What is something the adult you would tell your teenage self about your father-son relationship?
- How would your life be different today if you felt secure going into the world as a young man?
- What doubt or insecurity do you have about yourself as partner, man, friend, father, or employee?
- Did your father ever tell you that he was proud of you?
- Have you ever told your father that you love him?

The sense of feeling "not good enough" is the masculine crisis that every son must resolve in order to heal and develop a fulfilling life! Your father is part of your DNA, including your emotional makeup. Appreciating his strengths will allow you to see him more clearly.

Make no mistake: these questions are a gut check for the issues we buried many years ago under the mud of shame and anger. Now we are washing off the mud that has impaired, distorted, and psychologically blocked your ability to feel safe, to feel secure, and to be yourself.

Truly believing in your heart and soul that you are "defective" is toxic because you are not! The residual crippling emotions of your father factor, which undermine your confidence, cause you to question your masculinity, and hinder your love life, can change. Exposing these myths about yourself is the beginning steps of your healing process. The collateral damage of your past that was intrinsically created by the father-shaped wound inside of you is now expiring.

The deep sense of rejection that you have secretly carried in your soul is a lie. The goal of all psychological treatment modalities is to relieve your emotional pain and fears, healing the little boy trapped inside of you. The incredible burden of your father's shame

Gentlemen, your father-son story isn't going away because you choose to shelf it or kick it down the road.

has never been yours to shoulder or figure out. Your father's shame, inadequacies, personal fears, and distorted beliefs about himself and you don't have to remain hidden in your life. You aren't responsible for your father's healing; it's his journey to navigate.

This is the point in our story at which well-meaning, smart, and kind but fearful men run

A son personalizes his father's lack of support, love, and approval as a character flaw in himself, not as his father's lack of parenting!

from the prospect of peeling away the scar tissue from their father-son relationship. A common reaction to this prospect is to distract ourselves with everything else, with the unconscious intention of forever avoiding the visit to our father's house. A psychological truth is that no amount of money, career brilliance, public esteem, wealth, success, or accolades can heal what's inside of you. We have discussed in earlier chapters that our shame and "father wounds" are inside of us and must be handled from within.

> *When is a good time to stop running from yourself? You know the answer or you wouldn't be reading this book.*

The healing solution is to address the father-son fracture inwardly to end this male generational rejection cycle. The first step toward healing, mending, and strengthening your own sense of self and your "father factor" is consciously understanding the conscious and unconscious messages you learned growing up. This quote is a universal reminder that regardless of your background, ethnicity, trauma, culture, financial status, or emotional mood swings, the work of your healing starts within you. Anything else is simply postponing your personal masculine evolution.

> *There is nothing outside of yourself that can ever enable you to get better, stronger, richer, quicker, or smarter. Everything is within. Everything exists within. Seek nothing outside of yourself.*—Miyamoto Musashi

REWRITING DAD'S RULES FOR YOU—SPOKEN AND UNSPOKEN

Some of the important topics that all fathers and sons encounter in their lives are listed below. These rules are typically implied and understood without much explanation or reason. Often your father's rule book is the same one your grandfather gave him without question.

Write down the first thought you have regarding each of these subjects listed. One of the toughest personal challenges that men have in finding their own voice is understanding the unspoken rules that they are violating by not continuing to follow them, regardless of their usefulness or relevance. This is the book you read every day; what do you want to edit or keep?

Money
   Spoken:
   Unspoken:

Women/Sexuality
  Spoken:
  Unspoken:
Your Mother's Marriage and Divorce
  Spoken:
  Unspoken:
Work/Career Choices
  Spoken:
  Unspoken:
Morals/Ethics
  Spoken:
  Unspoken:
Mentoring/Fathering Style
  Spoken:
  Unspoken:
Health/Body Image
  Spoken:
  Unspoken:
Children/Family
  Spoken:
  Unspoken:
Failure/Loss/Disappointment
  Spoken:
  Unspoken:
Communication/Emotional Expression/Vulnerability
  Spoken:
  Unspoken:
Conflict Resolution
  Spoken:
  Unspoken:

YOUR RULE BOOK

Several things happen to young men as they enter their twenties and thirties. One is that they begin to question who is ultimately responsible for their choices. Fully embracing the consequences and responsibility for not making decisions and no longer blaming their fathers or others, this becomes the catalyst for the development of their road map of the next fifty years. Getting past the turbulent teen and college years, working full time, and beginning to enter the adult world, sons start to view their fathers differently, realizing that maybe their fathers weren't as out of it as they thought.

The quickest way to change is to take responsibility for what you aren't doing. Think about that.

Bumping against the guardrails of our fathers' intrinsic rules for himself and for you can be disorienting and scary. We have to pause and consider how to manage our career, marriage, finances, and masculinity. What are my priorities and my father's wishes for me?

Oftentimes, sons begin to see that dad, the "old man," isn't as stupid or outdated as they once thought. Sons meet other men who are the same age as their father and begin to realize that their dad isn't as odd or embarrassing as they thought.

MY DAD IS SOMEONE I DIDN'T KNOW

My client, Charlie, age twenty-five and a first-year attorney, met his father for lunch at Charlie's law firm in downtown Los Angeles. Charlie's boss, Fran, a senior partner at the firm, is the same age as his father (age fifty-six). Charlie introduced his father to Fran. A few hours later that day, Fran told Charlie that his father seemed like a good father and should be very proud of Charlie. Charlie told me this in our session: "Dr. P, I don't think I have ever viewed my father from the perspective of his peer group or what other fathers or men think of my Dad. I only hear my complaints about him and never considered that maybe he is a good man. I was surprised by how much my boss's comment affected me."

Boys naturally push away from their father figures; this is a process that they must master for their own autonomy. The elements of approval, acceptance, and love weave the fabric needed for their new psychological wardrobe and operating system. Lacking these invaluable pieces of their male identity can create resentful, rageful, and destructive young men. The rage of being or feeling neglected and lacking a sense of approval is psychologically devastating to the development of any type of positive emotional health, masculine strength, and life plan. Many boys angrily throw away their fathers' rule books and start down the path of self-destruction.

Fatherless sons have the emotional scars of feeling like "damage goods" as a result of not experiencing male acceptance, support, and understanding.

Not every social problem, gun violence issue, or mass murder crisis can be solved with healthier father-son relationships. Sons who have involved fathers don't carry the rage and explosive issues that fatherless sons experience. We know from years of research that boys who have involved fathers, positive father figures, and older male mentors live a different life than those boys lacking a masculine loving influence. Fatherless sons organically develop in reaction to their emotional deprivation, patterns of self-doubt, feelings of self-loathing, and poor choices. Angry boys grow up to be angry men who choose to get revenge against all authority and seek to hurt people the way that they have been damaged.

> *The quality of our life is directly connected to the emotional health of our relationship with ourselves and others!*

Sons start asking questions about why and how their fathers do what they do. Even if your dad died when you were very young or you never met him, his legacy was alive and well with your mother and the adults in your life. Sons of divorce wonder about their fathers, regardless of the marriage status or why the marriage ended. Sons want to know their fathers inside and out! Our masculine development is dramatically impacted and shaped by our father-son relationship. There is no way for a man to reach his full potential until he resolves and addresses his father-son relationship.

Sons will always want a relationship with their father in which they are seen, understood, and accepted. These three psychological building blocks are universal needs in all boys, at all ages. Men who never received their father's love and support many times turn their disappointment into anger and shame and then punish the world for their deep "father wound."

> *A man's masculinity will always include elements of his father-factor influence.*

NEW DAD STORY

Parker, age forty-two and a new client, is becoming a first-time father in a few months. Parker started to experience random panic attacks whenever he thought about having a newborn son. In our initial session, Parker told me:

> You know, I never met my dad. My parents separated when I was five months old. My mom and I moved a lot until I was eight years old, when she remarried a nice guy. I felt like I was my own father, since my dad was never around. I have had lots of male role models, mentors in my career and sports, and my stepfather, but being a father freaks me out.

How am I going to do it? I never thought I had any father issues until the last six months. I never thought my binge drinking and workaholic schedule had anything to do with my sadness. I now feel really sad that I never knew my father. I can't imagine ever leaving my son because my wife and I don't get along. This will not be my story or situation with my wife and children.

Even to this present day, twenty-first-century men, more times than not, look to their partners for emotional cues about how to relate to their children and for their emotional tools. Men, like women, are being pushed out of their comfort zones to embrace emotional equality.

Parker continued to resolve his repressed grief, anger, and feeling "defective" for never having had a father-son relationship. Parker did find tremendous comfort, support, and acceptance with his other father-son relationship (his stepfather). Parker was able to accept that although his biological father wasn't part of his life, it didn't diminish his ability to be the father he desires. His father-son relationship with his stepfather was the foundation that Parker built his fathering relationship on.

UNDERSTANDING OUR FATHERS

The importance of our emotional awakening for the psychological process of masculinity, mental health balance, and emotional intelligence are some of the reasons I pushed myself to write this book. Men want to be the father, partner, brother, son, friend, and man that their father wasn't able to be to them. This desire doesn't discount your father; rather, it's a heartfelt goal to do it differently. As men age, the rage and bitterness about their empty emotional connections, critical judgments regarding their careers, or being pushed to behave in certain ways begins to mellow. Sons emotionally soften when we begin to enter the world and see our fathers in the larger context of other men. There isn't the usual rage, resentment, and frustration with our fathers because sons (we are all sons) are beginning to see that their shortcomings were not deliberate or intentional. Men weren't expected or encouraged by the brotherhood to be emotionally available or insightful prior to the last twenty-five years. The tough-guy, emotionally disconnected, masculine model said, "That's the woman's role, not yours. Men aren't good with emotional stuff!" The majority of men I know personally and professionally—friends, colleagues, and clients—want to be the best version of themselves, not their father's version of masculinity.

Healthy masculinity embraces the ability to forgive, accept, and understand!

The problem, over the centuries and still at issue, is how to be emotionally intelligent, psychologically aware, and mentally connect with yourself and the important people in your life. The process of evolving emotionally and personal transformation is a lifelong journey with many rewards. Boys, regardless of age, unconsciously seek approval, acceptance, and love from their fathers—it's a natural biological drive. The challenge is that fathers like Brett's, Parker's, and mine were and are good men, but they just didn't have the tools to communicate their true feelings to us about life, women, careers, problem solving, positive communication, emotional expression, sex, marriage, vulnerability, finances, death, and the future.

Many men can't psychologically let go of their anger and resentment about their father's inability to be the father that they needed. We all know men who have spent a lifetime resenting their father and hating him to no avail. An Eastern spiritual psychological perspective on the futility of resentment is apropos: If you hate someone, dig two graves: one for the person you hate and another one for yourself.

What many boys, teenagers, young men, and grown men hate the most, both within and without, is their father and his neglect. Men try to ignore their hatred or become revengeful, because they don't know how to manage the raging river inside of them. Our fathers will always be part and parcel to who we are as men, fathers, husbands, colleagues, brothers, and uncles and who we are to ourselves, regardless of our age. Identifying with the parent of the same gender is a powerful bond that is unique to fathers and sons and mothers and daughters.

Let's just cut to the heart of the father-son relationship. The following items are psychological elements of every father-son relationship. It doesn't matter if your father went to prison for a violent crime or if he is a billionaire businessman, these issues are always present. Read the following statements and answer yes or no. I know this is difficult, but you already know the answers; let's be completely transparent with ourselves about our true feelings. This isn't the point in your journey to try to "cancel" or dismiss your father.

- *Love*—You know that you feel special to your father; emotionally you feel that you matter to him: *Yes or no*
- *Approval*—You are enough; you are psychologically and emotionally secure today. You don't seek other people's approval: *Yes or no*

- *Understanding*—You know who you are outside of your father's shadow; you have your own identity: *Yes or no*
- *Permission*—You live your own life; you are tolerant of differences between you and your father: *Yes or no*
- *Support*—Throughout your life, your father emotionally held you when you went into the world on your own: *Yes or no*
- *Kindness*—You understand yourself and your issues, and you choose not to judge your father or to create a self-loathing narrative about yourself (i.e., "I am bad," "This always happens to me," "My dad wasn't a good father."): *Yes or no*
- *Courage*—You are willing to try new things without knowing the outcome, and you instinctively have faith in your ability to land on your feet: *Yes or no*
- *Forgiveness*—You don't allow resentment, anger, or petty disagreements to influence your relationships; you have perspective, context, and understanding for your father's life and struggles: *Yes or no*
- *Individuality*—You actively find your own path without blaming others; you live independently of your father; you are responsible for your life, and you have the opportunity to build your life: *Yes or no*
- *Emotional boundaries*—You have the ability to tolerate frustration, anger, excitement and the ability to self-regulate impulses; you can say "No!" to important people in your life when necessary: *Yes or no*

Each of these elements comprise the substance of your mental health, psychological functioning, and the beginning of your masculinity. These ten variables are the building blocks to being the man you have always desired to be. The challenge is finding the balance for each of these inner personal variables for creating a fulfilling life.

RESOLVING YOUR RESENTMENT—MEETING AT DAD'S HOUSE

Here is how the story goes: Driving up to your father's house, your stomach tightens and you feel moderately anxious. You have come too far to stop now. You arrive and sit down in the living room and begin the talk.

What do you want to say to your father? This is your moment to untether yourself from the tyranny of anger and blame. Whatever it is that holds you back, you have the chance to unleash yourself from it. This is a scary moment of releasing the past and looking forward. All the physical abuse, emotional neglect, self-doubt, your parents' marriage/divorce, death(s), and abandonment is over!

Your father looks different than how you remember him. It's scary that he has aged and so have you. Maybe your father died years ago, and you realize that you get this imaginary chance to tell him what you have always wanted to tell him but the time had never been right. Now you can put aside your frustrations and let him know what he always meant to you deep down. You read the following letter to your father because you want him to know what you are thinking, feeling, and hoping to communicate.

Dear Dad,

I have always hoped we could have this opportunity to speak and . . .

Love,
[Your name]

We have to accept the possibility that true radiant energy in the male does not hide in, reside in, or wait for us in the feminine realm, nor in the macho/John Wayne realm, but in the magnetic field of the deep masculine.—Robert Bly, *Iron John: A Book about Men*

CHAPTER NINE

YOUR MOTHER FACTOR

Mom's Opinion of You and Your Masculinity

Attachment is indeed our most profound and foundational need!
—Ruth Cohn, marriage and family therapist

My mother is still mad at me for moving out of the house more than twenty-five years ago, getting married, and not being her emotional support system.—Evan, age forty-four

YOUR MOTHER—YOUR EMOTIONAL BAROMETER

Fully embracing one's masculinity requires an in-depth look at your mother's role in shaping your emotions, your relationship styles, and your ability to express your thoughts and feelings. We can't skip or avoid our mother's role in who and what we are as men. Our mothers' opinions of us and of our fathers carry a lot of weight in our view of masculinity. Yes, mom's perspective of men becomes our view of ourselves. For our mental health development as sons, it is invaluable that we become consciously aware of our mothers' feelings about and experiences with our fathers, grandfathers, uncles, and brothers. Your mother's feelings and experiences with and about men predates your birth. Your mother has her opinions, which are the emotional backdrop of your early years with her.

The mother-son relationship is special; it is not up for discussion or debate. In other words, our mothers are off-limits to everyone, including our wives and partners. This is sensitive, emotional material with lifelong residual influence, which most men dismiss.

> The first woman you ever loved was your mother! This fact makes your relationship with your mother the most prominent factor in your emotional development. Think about that.

Your relationship with your mother is sacred, and no one understands it better than you.

Guys will not argue this point—we know it's absolutely true—mothers help form our masculinity. No one criticizes our mother except us. The challenge is that we (me included) don't exactly know how to peacefully manage this all-encompassing relationship throughout our adult lives. When we disappoint her, the silent whisper in the back of our head says things like, "Well, she did give birth to you and took care of you growing up; do what she wants. She needs your attention."

A CAUTIONARY TALE—AN UNENDING STORY OF DESPAIR

This short story is a reminder that we must embrace all the aspects of our mother-factor to keep growing, healing, and becoming better men. Regardless of the conflicts, misunderstandings, resentments, disappointments, and emotional issues with our mother, we must look at the whole picture of who she is to us.

Evan, in one of the quotes opening this chapter, is discouraged that his mother seems resentful and bitter that Evan has a life beyond that of a responsible son; he's also a husband and father. Evan visited his mother in the hospital, where she was recuperating from her knee replacement, and she was caustic, sarcastic, and irritated with him. She admitted to Evan that she secretly never wanted him to move out or get married.

> My mom feels I don't take care of her like I should. She says that she feels abandoned by me for getting married and having kids. I tell my mother, "I have no idea what that means other than getting divorced and giving my teenagers away." She feels that I don't care about her. For the record, Dr. P., I was the only person in the family who came to see her!

While telling me this story, Evan throws his hands up in the air, exasperated by his mother's refusal to view him as an independent adult man rather than as her emotional husband. Evan's parents' marriage is cordial, emotionally distant, and lacking any passion or romance. Evan has felt responsible for his mother's happiness and emotional well-being for as long as he can remember. Evan acknowledged that his mother intended him to be successful and happy but never to leave her. The mixed message of love and abandonment has caused Evan to doubt his value in all his relationships.

This mother-son vignette is a common scenario for men when their mother-son attachment becomes the primary support system for the mother. When a son is raised by a mother who has unresolved emotional issues and childhood traumas, she sends the unspoken message: "never leave me." Young men struggle with this mixed message of becoming a man but staying close, never going too far away or leaving their mothers.

These emotional needs of the mother instinctively foster in the son a hyper-vigilant emotional radar system, and he becomes his mother's caretaker. Evan's story illustrates the push-pull separation process with his mother that his wife, Vicky, resents. Vicky dislikes Evan's mother's emotional dependency, chronic complaining, and manipulation of him.

One of the critical elements that men need for developing healthy relationships with women is the psychological ability to avoid seeking approval, rescuing women, and being codependent (i.e., losing your identity in the relationship). The unhealthy relationship dynamics of this style of mothering, when left unhealed, can cause the son to question his masculinity and create psychological confusion (i.e., emotional-physical boundaries) in all of his future relationships. How did Evan and his mother end up in an emotionally incestuous relationship? Before we answer this question, let's first explore how impactful, special, and important our mothers are to our emotional health and overall quality of life.

> *The mother-son relationship is where you learned how to understand your emotions and to regulate your feelings and moods.*

THE EMOTIONAL BEGINNINGS OF YOU AND MOM

Your initial bonding with your mother began during conception and continued through birth, toddlerhood, and on to the present day. It sounds odd to say, but we all started our story within our mothers' bodies. We shared her body, survived off her entire being via the umbilical cord. Many psychologists believe that there are two umbilical cords that must be severed between mother and son for their survival. First, the physical separation at birth. Second, emotional separation sometime between fifteen to twenty-five years old. Both of these experiences are critical to each individual's psychological mental health stability. Stop and seriously consider the mind-blowing concept that you and your mother shared the same body for nine months. As a result of this unique experience, you and your mother have a biological and emotional connection that's important to remember.

Then you, precious cargo, popped on the scene, screaming, and your male journey began. Your early years with your mother set the stage with the building blocks for your lifelong relationship style. Critical emotional tools that a son needs to master as he heads into adulthood are listed below. The mother-son bond sets the stage for our psychological, relational, and personal lifestyles choices and how we emotionally function in our adult world.

- *Style of emotional expression*—Expressing your feelings, thoughts, and ideas with words.
- *Intimacy-separation bonding*—Ability to tolerate leaving mom and coming back to her; psychologically secure; feeling secure when out of her presence. This bonding step teaches us how to be alone without feeling anxious, scared, or insecure about feeling loved.
- *Positive communication*—Non-shaming, encouraging feedback about your behavior, actions, and mistakes. You learn to articulate, describe, and express your feelings.
- *Personal boundaries*—Recognizing physical, emotional, verbal boundaries with yourself and others; knowing where you stop and start; physical and emotional space.
- *Fear of disappointment*—Unconditional support for learning; secure in your abilities about feeling loved and loving.
- *Misunderstandings with your mother and others*—Resolving conflict and still feeling loved when someone is upset; learning that feelings are temporary while maintaining psychological balance.
- *Psychological and physical needs*—Having your basic needs met via hugging, caregiving, and emotional attention. Your sense of having enough is a critical milestone.
- *Feeling valued*—Knowing you are special inside and out. You feel noticed and acknowledged for your intellectual and physical development.
- *Intangibles*—Nonverbal gestures of feeling supported, loved, and secure with your mom. These experiences of feeling "safe" were internalized as part of your expression of yourself. This included hugs and living life together emotionally connected.

MOTHER-FACTOR QUESTIONS ABOUT YOU

- Which of these psychological aspects listed above is lacking in your life?
- How do you feel when you are alone?
- What do you fear?

- What area of your life do you feel self-doubt?
- How do you create boundaries in your relationships?
- How do you express your anger?
- What makes you feel loved?
- How uncomfortable are you when someone is upset with you?
- Who gave you a sense of approval growing up?
- What is something you need/want in your love/romantic/marriage relationship?
- How do you handle uncomfortable feelings?
- How do you show feelings of love/affection?

Voluminous dissertations have been written on each of the topics listed above. This is a quick overview of some of the intricate psychological pieces that impact your life. The items listed above are outlines that illustrate your mother's enormous role in setting the stage for your relationship style/attachment style with her. The differences in this relationship compared with your relationship with your father in no way diminishes either parent. We are not choosing one parent over the other or grading their value in your development. Your relationship with your parents simply points out the incredible importance that these two people have had in your masculine formation, your mental health, your quality-of-life choices, your career decisions, and whom and why you marry. We discuss two important bookends in your life. We aren't cancelling your parents, but rather gaining a wider perspective of who they are and their value in shaping you.

> *The mother-son relationship is the psychological blueprint of a man's ability to be emotionally vulnerable and self-regulated!*

Mothers, mothering, and your mother-son bond has been a subject of psychology since the beginning of time. Human history has always held a special place for mothers, which has been rightfully earned. Mothers have always had the responsibility to nurture the kids, produce life, and manage the family's emotional health. This is still true today; now both parents are expected to help inside the house and outside the house. It's a challenging task for mothers and fathers, married adults, and single adults with or without kids to juggle all these different gender roles. The task of nurturing, parenting, and caring for elderly parents, maintaining our intimate relationships, working, living, and simultaneously managing our own life is a nonstop process.

The following questions are true or false—you know if you use and experience these basic relationship tools growing up.

- *You were allowed to express yourself*—You felt emotionally secure to express yourself, and your opinion, wants, and ideas were valued: *True or false?*
- *You received daily attention*—Your physical health, emotional mood swings, and educational needs were important: *True or false?*
- *You received physical affection*—You were physically hugged and held as a young child, and you were "noticed" when you came home by your mother and your family: *True or false?*
- *Your home was predictable*—Your home life was stable (not perfect), with normal ups and downs, and you felt physically safe: *True or false?*
- *Your family felt emotionally safe*—You weren't scared or abused by your siblings or relatives: *True or false?*

The intangibles of the mother-son relationship are the unconscious template that you use in your relationships, marriage/romance, experiencing feelings, emotional problem-solving skills, and expressing affection verbally, emotionally, and physically. Men either underestimate or overestimate the magnitude of their mother's "hand" in creating our psychological-emotional hardwiring.

> *How we perceive, feel, and think about ourselves emotionally today began with our mother-son verbal and nonverbal communication.*

Developmental psychologists say that the way our mother spoke to us in our childhood is the psychological foundation of our perception of either feeling competent or inferior by the age of five. *The internal picture we carry around of ourselves is handcrafted in this one-of-a-kind relationship.* We learn from firsthand experience our emotional "man skills" in navigating female/male intimate relationships, being vulnerable when feeling sad or loving, having insight into ourselves and others.

We automatically internalize how our mother felt about us growing up. During our childhood and adolescent years, the formation of our sense of self is directly related to the quality of our mother/son emotional connection. This relationship started in the womb and evolved into our inner narrative about how we feel about being around our siblings and childhood friends.

When these basic tasks are incomplete, disrupted, and not fully understood, the son's emotional wounds begin. Throughout history, the discussions about mothers often

> *The basic life skills of becoming a kind, courageous, emotionally stable, high-functioning, and responsible man are the fundamental tasks of the mother-son dance.*

relate to the problems created when these important life tasks for the son get derailed. It's possible to pinpoint when emotional fractures occurred in your relationship with your mother. The damaging side effects of this relationship going awry shed light into how wounded boys become dangerous men. Healing these early emotional disappointments allows you to experience your full expression of yourself and your masculinity.

MOTHER FACTOR DEFINED

The questions above are designed to help you recall some of the emotional memories you carry with you today. Many of the personality traits, fears, emotional strengths, relationship balance, and life goals have their beginnings in the first ten years of life.

Let's get into the deep end of your mother's influence on you and understand the magnitude of your mother factor. The working definition for this all-important relationship in your life that we use is as follows:

> Your emotional development, functioning, and ability to form meaningful relationships in your family, in all areas of your life, and with intimate partners; an emotional template beginning with your mother-son bond that impacts your feelings of frustration, love, fear, and hope; your mother's style of parenting as the model for your emotional disposition and your core sense of who and what you are in the world; your emotional functioning as consciously and unconsciously shaped by your mother's attachment to you. (See Stephan Poulter's *Mother Factor: How Your Mother's Emotional Legacy Impacts Your Life*.)

MOTHER-FACTOR QUESTIONS
(BE HONEST—SHE ISN'T READING THEM!)

- What are some of your early (before age ten) memories of your mother?
- What is your first thought or feeling you have about your childhood?
- How would describe your relationship with your mom growing up: stable and predictable or unstable?
- As a child, did you feel liked by your mother?
- Do you like your mother today?
- Do you remember being hugged as a child?
- What is something that you appreciate about your mother?
- What is one of your mother's strengths, talents, or gifts?
- How did you and your mother handle disagreements?

- What is the emotional picture you carry of your mother in your heart?
- Did your mother like your father?

These questions are intended to help you recall some of your important memories and forgotten childhood stories—not all positive or all negative. I know it's difficult to discuss a traumatic abusive mother-son relationship. These questions wash away some of the layers of mud that has accumulated on your inner gold brick—your inner pure self. You are now exposing the mud shame that has blocked you with anger, frustration, and confusion. All your steps to heal, understand, and develop a positive masculinity allow you to experience new degrees of fulfillment and peace of mind.

The actual day-to-day experience of your mother factor was played out within your relationship-style attachment between you and your mom. I know there is a lot of material about attachment styles in the popular media, which is valuable. We explore your mother's attachment style in chapter 11, which explains her relationship style.

A secure relationship is exemplified in the ways that your mother emotionally connected and physically bonded with you (hugs), the tone of voice she used when talking to you, and how she nurtured you when you were upset or sick. The psychological, emotional, social, and educational parts of you were engaged in this day-to-day process. This is why you and your mother's relationship is so critical to comprehend! It is like dissecting blood cells: the closer you look, the more you discover. This applies to your relationship with your mother.

> *Adult sons' feelings about their mothers are a good indicator of their overall emotional functioning and mental health.*

Are you starting to see that your relationship challenges with your partner and work colleagues, your financial pressures, and your health issues aren't in a vacuum? It's all related, connected, and blended together in how you manage your life today. Oftentimes we are so close to the problem that we don't see the answer. Because we are the answer—never forget that! Your masculine expression encompasses all of these different emotional pieces of you, which come together to form your approach to the people in your life and your mental health balance.

THE EMOTIONAL ATMOSPHERE OF YOUR CHILDHOOD

We're so repressed emotionally. Just look at how many people apologize for crying!—Dr. Nicole Le Pera, psychologist

Getting Out of Your Own Way

Men need healing! Men need to let go and never again use the tough-guy macho-bravado mask as a means of coping with life. Emotional illiteracy is a deliberate choice to avoid learning how to read your own psychology—how you emotionally understand yourself and others. Earlier in the book, we discussed that your emotional intelligence starts with being vulnerable. Learning to decode your emotional language is your superpower. This requires reading and knowing your emotional mood swings, reactions, and feelings.

For example, seemingly friendly adult men who want to remain emotionally in the dark become defensive when they find out that I am a psychologist. Some guys spontaneously tell me that they don't believe in therapy or that it's for mentally ill people. Trying not to be irritated by

Bullies are secretly scared of the terror that lies within them!

their passive-aggressive statement, my response goes something like this: "I didn't know that therapy was a belief system rather than a personal growth experience. What's wrong with men wanting to be better fathers, husbands, friends, colleagues, or sons? It takes courage to explore self-improvement, personal growth, and the desire to improve their life!"

Usually, the topic is dropped, and the discussion goes in another direction. Such remarks aren't about believing or not believing in therapy but the terror that lies within the men who make those comments. This type of male bullying via humor isn't humor but a sign of unresolved mother-son issues.

When we choose to remain emotionally stuck, resisting change, this relationship style disrupts all our relationships. The pattern of avoidance limits our emotional intelligence. Avoiding, dismissing, mocking, bullying those men who embrace their manhood is no longer acceptable for adult men to do or to allow others to do. Covering up the pain stored within is the formula for self-loathing, living in constant fear. We men can allow ourselves to feel our feelings; it will not kill us to do it.

Emotional illiteracy is a choice to remain disconnected from your feelings, emotions, and their impact on others and your life.

Just ask a man what he loves to do or what team he loves to watch. Then tell him it's not good and he shouldn't or can't do it any longer. You will get a visceral, passionate, enthusiastic response defending his interests. These same talents and abilities to articulate his feelings are transferable to our relationships and intimate partners.

Evan, who we met earlier in the chapter, related a story about the embarrassment and shame he feels about his relationship with his mother. Evan told me the following:

> Recently I told my mom that I can't take her out for dinner or brunch every weekend. Second, I told her to stop texting me every day, checking up on me to make sure I am okay. She became very angry, accusing me of cutting her out of my life. I lost my temper and screamed at her that I am not her boyfriend. My mother said, "It feels like you are breaking up with me, and good sons don't do that to their mother." I stopped talking to her and hung up.

While relating this story to me, Evan started feeling guilty and doubting himself: setting limits with his mother is mean. Evan said that when he feels rageful frustration, he plays video games for hours to numb out. Four or five hours later, Evan can breathe again and calm down. These episodes are scary but happen less frequently since Evan no longer avoids his resentment and anger regarding this situation. Evan loves his mother but dislikes her when she tries to manipulate him with guilt.

You can love someone and not like them at the same time!

TAKING ACTION FOR YOUR BEST SELF

Men come to therapy to feel better. We want to unburden our secret traumas and gain some emotional relief from our inner critics. Men know that the pathway begins with shedding healing tears of sorrow about their traumas and disappointments suppressed in their hearts and souls.

For instance, Brent, a forty-year-old father, had to discuss the pedophile sports coach who molested Brent's friends, though everyone else pretended it didn't happen and never talked about it. Peter, twenty-six years old, needed to discuss his weird male cousin who always tried to isolate Peter's younger sister in the bedroom whenever the families got together. He threatened to kill Peter if he ever told anyone. At the time, the cousin was sixteen years old, Peter was eight, and his sister was six years old; no one would have believed Peter if he had said something. Peter's cousin was ultimately hospitalized for a delusional thought disorder and is now under psychiatric care.

As young men, we didn't know what to do with these troubling situations. Compounding it, we are frustrated about bottling up all this pain. Confusion and impending doom are feelings we rigorously attempt to avoid. As young boys, we couldn't articulate our feelings and thoughts or voice contrary opinions. If we did speak up, the old-school male bully machine would flatten our hearts and souls. If we didn't talk about what was going on at home, then things felt better outside the house. Our moms seemed distant, distracted, or anxious. Our fathers were around but not emotionally engaged, or they lived somewhere else. We didn't want to upset our parents, so we stayed silent with our thoughts and worries.

> *Growth demands a temporary surrender of security.*—Gail Sheehy, author

HOW DO I START DISCUSSING *MY* FEELINGS

Sadness, terror, depression, anxiety, addictive impulses, forgiveness, kindness, compassion, and hope are emotions we desperately need to become more familiar with. This isn't "psychobabble"; we are opening up our man caves and finally discussing our childhood challenges. Old nonverbal habits of looking for answers outwardly instead of inwardly have run their course, offering no relief or solutions. Men working nonstop, making huge amounts of money, and being constantly on the go are all well-designed plans for avoiding our unresolved, unprocessed, and unedited childhood/adult struggles.

We have buried the memories, the pain, the powerlessness, and the helplessness. Well, those issues tend to reappear at the most inopportune time in your life, as discussed earlier in the book.

Now is the time to stop, pause, and reexamine our psychological-emotional hard drives for healing purposes. This is how we are going to turn things around and improve our lives and circles of influence. Angry men and reckless boys have one thing in common—they are both secretly looking for a supportive father figure. Men who understand their childhood emotional strengths and deficits will stop punishing the women in their life. Domestic violence started in the abuser's childhood home and within the parental relationship—this is an unfortunate fact. Men who feel secure, content, and good about themselves don't abuse their partners or the people around them—they don't need to! If you are a victim or abuser, this is the time to pause and stop this cycle of self-hatred.

The women or men we love, know, support, and believe in have nothing to do with our mother- and father-factor wounds. Our mothers began our

Shame tells us that we are damaged goods incapable of changing.

emotional learning processes at home. Our fathers showed us how to function in the world, not to punish the world. Now it's time for us to finish our education, taking full responsibility for our lives, our relationships, and actions. Don't allow your shame, guilt, or despair to prevent you from starting to resolve and heal your inner self! Remember, shame lies and says things are "hopeless." It's never hopeless, never!

FOUR EMOTIONAL HEALING STEPS TO TAKE TODAY—OUR LIFELINE

- *Accepting what happened*, not the watered-down version—no denial
- *Grieving* the scared, confused, neglected boy inside of you
- *Resolving your trauma* with new emotional limits and insights
- *Writing a new script* for your life going forward—literally and figuratively

I explain how to actively engage these four action steps for washing away your emotional mud while gaining clarity and resolution. Entering the dark, unspoken emotions of fear and self-loathing is the only way that terror and shame stay alive inside of you. Many of our mental roadblocks and emotional missteps had their genesis in the emotional climate between you and your mother. Psychologists have illuminated the importance of the mother-infant bond as a template for the child's future relationships personally, romantically, and socially. I discuss your father's role in your healing process in the next two chapters.

Again, this isn't a blaming or mother-bashing session. We look at the good, the bad, and the ugly of *you*. It takes courage to be honest and transparent about our physical, emotional, relational, and mental health. Blaming your mother for all your challenges is like drinking poison and hoping it kills the other person. It's worth repeating: if you are angry and want to blame your mother for what she did or didn't do correctly in your life, just know you will not find any peace of mind or happiness.

TRANSLATING OUR FEELINGS, THOUGHTS, AND ACTIONS

What Does Acceptance Mean, and How Does It Work for Me?

The act of acceptance is acknowledging what happened in your life without covering it up with emotion. This requires a cognitive-intellectual look at what "really" happened, not what you wanted or thought happened. Abuse is a topic for men that gets very little attention, because men feel humiliated for admitting that something happened in the past that was not appropriate—you know if things were right or not right! We men must address our experience of abuse—verbal, emotional, physical, and sexual.

How Do I Grieve for Myself?

This is a great question because it requires you to visualize the little boy inside of you. Try to remember how it felt growing up when things weren't good: when life was turbulent with your parents, or your brother died, or you got cancer. Grieving is acknowledging, as an adult, that the little person inside of you needed someone to hold and understand him. Grieving is allowing the emotions of that day when you got the news that your mother died in a car accident, or your parents were getting a divorce, or your best friend moved across the country. Many times, our first experience of loss is when our childhood pet dies—it's devastating for boys at any age. Grieve for things that you lost or left in your life. Grief isn't a pity party; it's uncovering your heartbreaks.

How Do I Resolve My Trauma?

The best way I know how to explain this three-dimensional process on paper is that you must leave the past in the past using your adult insights, strength, and memory. It's important to remember that you are not a helpless ten-year-old boy getting beaten or molested. You are an adult man with resources, knowledge, and abilities to take care of yourself today. You will never be a child again or powerless to protect and take care of yourself. The key is not allowing your past trauma to control your present-day life with fear, anxiety, and impending doom. This isn't having amnesia about your past abuse but putting it on the bookshelf of your life. Your life is not replaying the helplessness of the past every time you get upset or feel vulnerable. Your past wounds, fears, and childhood behaviors are not controlling your adult life.

How Do I Write a New Script for My Life?

The first step is realizing that a script already exists. Whether you know it or not, there is a script unconsciously and consciously influencing your life. You have to find this script, who wrote it, what the storylines are, how the lead actor (you) handles life, relationships, work, children, parents, money, health, success, body image, siblings, divorce, and disappointments. All these variables are in your script and have great importance for your healing going forward. You are completely in control of how you want to rewrite the script of your life with positive outcomes, success, and fulfillment.

START YOUR NEW SCRIPT WITH THESE PERSONAL QUESTIONS

- What is something that is difficult to accept about myself or about my childhood?
- What is something that makes me really sad whenever I think of my mother?
- How do I resolve my trauma from twenty years ago?
- What is something that I am holding on to from my past that is holding me back today?
- What is my life plan, my script for the things I desire and want to do?

> *Most people never heal, because they stay in their heads replaying corrupted scenarios. Let it go.* —S. McNutt

CHAPTER TEN

MASCULINITY, CONNECTION, AND YOUR STYLE OF RELATIONSHIPS

Creating Emotional Stability

Your relationship with yourself sets the tone for every other relationship you have.—Robert Holden

And God said, "Love Your Enemy," and I obeyed him and loved myself.—Kahlil Gibran, poet

Finding a stable love when all you knew growing up was chaos is one of the most under-recognized achievements. The love you can count on, the love you wake up in the middle of the night to laugh with, the love that feels like home should have always been felt.—Dr. Nicole LePera, clinical psychologist

Please all, and you will please none.—Aziz Hubbard

YOUR OWN STYLE OF CONNECTING— A LIFELONG ADVENTURE

We have discussed a wide range of subjects surrounding our masculinity, emotional life, health, upbringing, parents, sexuality, emotional intelligence, healing childhood traumas, physical appearance, therapy, and now your love life! The subjects of men, dating, sex, friendships with "benefits," female-male sensuality, and romance are endless for both men and women of all ages. When in doubt, ask someone about their love life, and you definitely will generate some talking points.

Over the years in my psychological practice, I've learned that men of all ages—starting at age eight to age ninety—are trying to find romantic relationships, ending romantic relationships, considering marriage, maintaining their marriage, or managing the disillusionment of their former marriage. Men and relationships, with whatever gender you are attracted to, are opportunities for full emotional expression, self-acceptance, and transparency of who you are and who you desire to be. Masculinity is the cement floor upon which our attachment and relationship styles are built. Your masculine expression is the way that you connect and feel in all your various types of relationships.

A Cautionary Tale—Placating the Family

Jackson, a kind, emotionally predictable, thoughtful, caring adult, husband, and father, is his dad's business partner in their real estate company. Jackson has a gentle spirit and a strong backbone. Jackson is personable, accommodating, and a "fixer" for his childhood family, his friends, his business, and his wife. At first glance, Jackson seems like a caring man who likes to help everyone. Taking a closer look below the surface of Jackson's relationship style, many of his behaviors are coping mechanisms stemming from his chaotic childhood. Publicly Jackson presents the perfect picture of mental health, but he is a neglected soul who had to learn how to adapt his attachment style to psychologically compensate for his chaotic and emotionally volatile family. Jackson's masculine development was shaped by having to tend to his own needs and wants as a child because of the marital tension between his parents.

Our natural attachment drive and the need for it never diminishes throughout our life—never.

Attaching, bonding, and connecting to the various people in our relationships is how our personality emerges. Our character, values, personal emotional needs, and who we are privately and publicly are all related and inseparable. Other words, your personal and professional priorities, important attachments (people, possessions), emotional connections (family, institutions), and types of relationships (work, social) are a picture board of you.

Another hot topic concerning men is our ability (or inability) to form short- and long-term relationship commitments, to remain faithful emotionally or physically, and to maintain secure, trusting partnerships personally, professionally, and socially. These subjects are different combinations of your attachments, degrees of vulnerability, and important relationships.

Before we charge into men and romantic relationships, there are two things we need to establish. First, how do you attach, connect, and emotionally express yourself? Second, what is your type or style of relationship? These two variables work hand in hand to form your ability to psychologically, emotionally, mentally, socially, and physically connect with others and to experience meaningful relationships. The framework is your relationship style. Both of these processes are part of your unique personality expression. Who, what, why, and how you are in relationships has been "in process" since your birth.

During the first three years of your life, bonding to your mother was as significant as eating, sleeping, and learning to walk! Do you know (you can ask your family) if the first three years of your life were calm, peaceful, and stable or chaotic and unpredictable for your mom?

As an infant you reflexively attached to your mother, which was your first experience of love and frustration.

How was her pregnancy with you and your early childhood? The reason is that developmental psychologists attribute many of our adult personality problems to difficult times that our mothers experienced during our early bonding years. Your mother's state of mind—whatever that might have been—during your early experiences of having your needs met in a regular, predictable, and stable manner set the stage for how you experience adult relationships.

The psychological wellness of our moms during our formative years is a major element of our mental health and emotional wants in intimate relationships as adult men. These all-important issues surrounding the mother-son relationship are why so much has been written about this very special time in a child's and mother's life. Your initial experiences of physical satisfaction (being fed), emotional satisfaction (being held), and psychological stability (reassurance that you are safe) with your mother during your childhood can't be emphasized enough. Don't be alarmed if your early years were anything but calm; you can overcome your early psychological disappointments.

WHY YOUR ATTACHMENT STYLE MATTERS— DESPAIR VERSUS CONTENTMENT

I can't reiterate how many of my clients' relationship issues are recycled! No one wants to hear this, but it's true and early childhood research supports the fact that your early emotional bond with your mother is vital to your development. You will project your unresolved emotional needs with your mother onto your current romantic partner. Often my male clients point their fingers at their partners, believing that they are at fault for the men's emotional struggles. They firmly believe that the emotionally withholding, emotionally distant, demanding women/partners they are dating or married to have to be the

The majority of your personal issues predate the problems recycling in your current relationship; they are old, unresolved themes.

problem in the relationship. Men who struggle with intimacy, anger, depression, or feeling unlovable or unimportant to their partners are dealing with issues that predate all of their relationships! Read this sentence again.

The underlying relationship problem began early in your life: not having your needs noticed or met, feeling misunderstood and unsafe during your childhood. These mother-son interactions created your psychological sense of deprivation as a young boy and automatically replay today in your attachment and relationship patterns. This is why our masculinity development will never be fully actualized until we go inward and address our unspoken needs and wants. Money, success, material possessions, or career importance will not heal the needy young boy inside of you. Your external accomplishments are wonderful, impressive, and noteworthy, but they are incapable of fixing what's within.

Changing your reoccurring attachment/relationship patterns of feeling frustration and having unmet emotional needs starts with recognizing the longstanding nature of these feelings and experiences. Be mindful that your early childhood connections to your mother and father were not always fully

Attachment theory premise: Our first bonding experience has the power to unconsciously set expectations for all our subsequent relationships!

operational. This doesn't imply that your childhood was a disaster, a dumpster fire, or terrible. No parent (me included) can be perfect, the ideal nurturer emotionally connected to you all the time. In the field of psychology, mental health problems are evaluated in degrees of severity, repetition, and levels of impairment. Perfection isn't a measurement of mental health; it's viewed as an emotional defense mechanism against feeling shameful and defective.

You might have been sad periodically as a boy, but that doesn't mean your childhood predisposed you to adult depression today. Let's ask and answer some questions about your attachment history with your parents.

Attachment Questions—You and Your Parents

The list below is a sampling of interactions, behaviors, and feelings that occur throughout our lives. Be aware as you read the list that some behaviors are ongoing. The emotional mood in your childhood and present day is important to understanding your mental health today. Do the best you can to recall, feel, and picture the little boy within along with the male adult answering these questions.

Your Attachment Style

- You have difficulty trusting and emotionally connecting with friends, colleagues, and family members. *Yes or no?*
- You have been told that you are aloof and that it is difficult to know you socially, professionally, and intimately. *Yes or no?*
- You don't like hugging, cuddling, or being touched by friends or your romantic partner. *Yes or no?*
- You don't like strong emotional expressions. *Yes or no?*
- You respected both your parents, regardless of their marriage status. *Yes or no?*
- You are ambivalent about keeping "in touch" with your friends. *Yes or no?*
- You have new and long-term significant male relationships. *Yes or no?*
- You express strong feelings of appreciation to coworkers, friends, and your romantic partner. *Yes or no?*
- You are able to resolve or minimize personality conflicts at work, home, and personally. *Yes or no?*
- You avoid interacting with people whenever possible. *Yes or no?*
- You have difficulty expressing contrary opinions to your boss, close friends, partner, and family. *Yes or no?*
- You are comfortable with having psychological closure with people, job changes, and moving away. *Yes or no?*

Your Mother's Attachment Style with You

- Your mother didn't emotionally engage with you as child. *Yes or no?*
- Your mother could read your emotions when you walked into the house and would engage you. *Yes or no?*
- Your mother would become angry and verbally aggressive toward you. *Yes or no?*
- Your mother blamed you for her lack of professional success. *Yes or no?*
- You felt special and nurtured by your mother. *Yes or no?*
- You knew your mother always loved you, in spite of your mistakes and behaving poorly at times. *Yes or no?*
- Your mother respected your father. *Yes or no?*

- Your mother didn't play favorites with you or your siblings. *Yes or no?*
- Your mother was interested in everything you did or tried. *Yes or no?*
- Your mother felt emotionally safe, predictable, and patient. *Yes or no?*

Your Father's Attachment Style with You

- Your father never expressed joy or happiness about being your father. *Yes or no?*
- Your father resented working in a career/job that made money for the family rather than following his passion. *Yes or no?*
- You knew that your father loved and adored you. *Yes or no?*
- Your father was emotionally distant. *Yes or no?*
- Your father spent time with you. *Yes or no?*
- Your father respected your mother and women. *Yes or no?*
- Your father could emotionally regulate his moods, impulses, and anger. *Yes or no?*
- Your father struggled with alcohol use and being moody. *Yes or no?*
- Your father hugged you. *Yes or no?*
- Your father did not express strong emotions or feelings. *Yes or no?*

If most of your responses to these three lists of questions are "yes," then you most likely experienced a secure, stable style of attachment with both your parents. It is more common to experience attachment relationship issues with one parent than with both of your parents. Oftentimes one parent is distant and the other parent overcompensates for them, which doesn't feel natural to you. The extent to which you recognize that you have personal issues with one or both of your parents is the same extent to which you can resolve those issues. Healing and acceptance are directly related and complementary. The truth is that you can resolve and create meaningful connections and secure stable relationships. Many times, we aren't fully aware of the "learned" way that we make friends, meet people, and interact with others until we experience some type of major romantic heartbreak, loss of a close buddy, or falling out with a childhood friend. These relationship breakdowns and transitions often highlight our emotional blind spots.

Women Know Attachment

Attachment theory is becoming increasingly more popular as a mainstream concept, a natural process between a mother and baby, and for good reason.

Attachment, bonding, and these types of psychological, emotional, physical, social, and career connections provide deep human meaning, informing us of who and what we are and where and how we impact the world. Women know this fact and have been connecting together for centuries. There are good reasons why groups like "Mommy and Me," a mother-infant group, meet and form lifelong friendships among their members, who have children of the same age. Women's book clubs, for instance, often meet for many years because of the psychological value of being with other likeminded women. Men are beginning to realize the wealth and value of emotionally supportive male friends. Old-school masculinity is based on isolation, without emotional expression or vulnerability. This model has never been viable or productive for forming fulfilling male relationships.

> **Mental health is based on our ability to establish and maintain secure relationships.**

The value, meaning, and experience of life comes through the avenue of our attachments, which is our relationship lifeblood. The absence of these vital bonds, meaningful attachments, and feelings of belonging are detrimental to our overall health and psychological stability. In severe situations of isolation, the absence of emotional relationships can become fatal (suicide). Over time, lacking relationship bonds, young boys start to emotionally withdraw from the outside world.

These boys are psychologically guarded against the feelings of frustration and powerlessness of their parent-child bonds. When men begin to dismantle their emotional blocks, which were created from years of empathic failures (a pattern of no one noticing your needs), good things happen.

Your Own Attachment Styles

Now let's talk about the guru of attachment theory, Dr. John Bowlby, a famous British psychiatrist who brought his in-depth research on the lifelong importance of attachment to the mental health community. Prior to Dr. Bowlby's findings during the early 1950s, attachment theory was a secondary concern for the psychological health of children. Fortunately, during the last seventy-five years, the invaluable importance of a child's ability to emotionally attach is now considered one of the primary tasks for all young children. Many mental illness diagnoses are attributed to a child's early years of emotional disruption within the mother-child attachment process and an unpredictable relationship.

Here we discuss Dr. Bowlby's five basic styles of attachment, which every son develops naturally as a result of the emotional and relational environment in which he was raised from birth to age five. The child (you) organically adapts to the strengths and weakness of his caretakers, parents, and home environment. The five styles are as follows: intermittent (random), avoidant (distant), anxious (overwhelmed and overwhelming), depressed (lacking energy and focus), and secure (consistent).

You may have elements of all five styles simultaneously, but you will have one predominate pattern of relating. We blend and use our primary attachment style along with the other four patterns in our friendships, acquaintanceships, and our social, family, and personal relationships.

INTERMITTENT (RANDOM) STYLE OF ATTACHMENT

The name implies the hit-or-miss, inconsistent, and unpredictable nature of the mother's mood swings, distractions, anxiety, and natural reluctance to remain fully bonded with her son. The relationship is unpredictable, and it is very confusing for the young child. The underlying reasons for mothers' erratic behavior are that her unmet emotional and relational needs interfere with her ability to fully focus on parenting. The random-attachment mother is not emotionally engaged and is unaware of or does not notice her sons' normal ups and downs of life.

There is an inconsistent focus—distraction, lack of attention to details, and then a hyperfocus—on the sons' lives. There is no pattern to this mother focus and attention, and it is very troubling for her son, who can't trust or feel safe with her.

For instance, the second grader needs his field trip slip signed and paid for. The mother misses the email, and the boy is the only child in his class who can't go on the field trip. Two weeks later, the same mother volunteers for the school's spring carnival, organizes other volunteers to help, and is fully involved in her son's life that week.

Unfortunately, the infrequent emotional attention eventually creates a lack of trust in the child himself and in his mother. This young boy begins to feel and experience that his world isn't a safe place, that no one cares or notices him. This core wounding follows him into adulthood: the world and people aren't safe. The consistent mother instills in her son trust that she does care and that good things happen in his life. The random mother *unintentionally* creates and reinforces in her son's early life experiences that things aren't fair and that bad things happen to him.

This boy often grows up to become pessimistic, sarcastic, and cynical about life and love. The good things of life—positive feelings and nice friendships—seem to escape or evade this boy-man unconsciously; he is unaware that he has created a protective emotional shell over his painful childhood neglect. This man tends to interpret personal and professional friendships and situations negatively. All of these self-protective behaviors form and shape his masculinity through a negative view of himself and life. Beneath his tough exterior is an emotional pool of bitterness, disappointment, and sadness drowning his best self.

Please remember that new insights will bring positive changes in your life. It's very painful to look within, at how we became sad and lonely. All the topics in this book, including this one, are amenable to positive change, healing, and transforming your life from within.

Do I Have Intermittent (Random) Tendencies?

- You find it difficult to sincerely trust my colleagues, friends, and intimate partners. *Yes or no?*
- You emotionally withdraw and shut down when you are upset, hurt, sad, or frustrated. *Yes or no?*
- You consider yourself to be cynical or have a pessimistic view of your world. *Yes or no?*
- You confide in a friend, coworker, or partner, about your feelings, fears, and hopes? *Yes or no?*
- You believe that people in your life truly care and love you. *Yes or no?*
- You avoid emotionally charged situations and emotionally expressive people. *Yes or no?*
- You consider yourself a loner, preferring to be by yourself than with people. *Yes or no?*

The more "yes" answers to these questions—your thoughts about your capacity and desire for emotional intimacy—might signal that you are emotionally intermittent in your relationships. Insights concerning your psychological development being influenced by the inconsistent attachment pattern of your mother can be the catalyst for changing all your relationships.

AVOIDANT (DISTANT) STYLE OF ATTACHMENT

The avoidant-attaching mother was not emotionally expressive or interested in that form of connection. There wasn't any type of warm, embracing communication with feeling or excitement. The avoidant style of attaching is cerebral, absent of emotional intelligence, and stoic. There is a lack of energy in the mother-son bond. The relationship is functional, not loving. Emotions, feelings, passion, and excitement are high-energy exchanges that weren't part of this relationship. Hugging, hand-holding, bedtime rituals, and other types of nurturing behaviors also weren't elements in this relationship. These acts of emotional distance, aloofness, and noncommunicative feelings leave the boy feeling incomplete, lacking in himself. The mother discounts any type of psychological explanation for her son's inability to express feelings and emotional issues. There is a very clear unspoken emotional distance between the mother and son at all times, regardless of any situation.

This mother was responsible, thorough, and caring. Mom loves her son but doesn't say it or communicate it in any type of empathic way—it's not her style. Over time, this boy feels isolated and emotionally empty. For example, the son comes home after school and learns that his dog was hit by a car. The boy starts crying, and the mother says "sorry" and walks into the other room. This child is left with feelings of embarrassment about crying even though it's an appropriate reaction to important relationship loss. The unspoken message is that close emotional attachments are dangerous, keep your distance to be safe.

A lack of self-confidence combined with self-doubt and being a loner make forming friendships and emotional interactions tremendously difficult to do. You are viewed as an outsider in your peer group. It feels unnatural to be emotional or to express your feelings—it is like a foreign language to you and not your first response or reaction to important events, situations, or sadness. You feel awkward trying to understand social and emotional cues from people. Your attachment issues are not neurologically based, such as with autism or Asperger's syndrome.

> *Emotional connections are unsafe and should be avoided whenever possible.*

Your emotional blocks are issues from your childhood, not a reflection of your capacity to change or become emotionally engaged. The absence of social and emotional skills with which to connect with people seems normal to you. Attachment for this adult son is cognitive, not emotionally experienced or heartfelt.

Do I Have Avoidant (Distant) Tendencies?

- You are frequently told that you are in your "head" and emotionally distant from the conversation, people, or event. *Yes or no?*
- You struggle with being emotionally vulnerable with close friends, colleagues, and your family. *Yes or no?*

- You have difficulty maintaining close contact with people. *Yes or no?*
- Any type of strong emotion or feelings makes you uncomfortable? *Yes or no?*
- You avoid your friends and social gatherings. *Yes or no?*
- Your family and partner feel that you are aloof and tend to be "cold" and impersonal. *Yes or no?*
- Reading peoples' nonverbal communication is problematic for you. *Yes or no?*
- You prefer to have casual friendships because of the familiarity and comfort level. *Yes or no?*
- People don't consider you to be a warm and caring person, even though you care deeply about people. *Yes or no?*
- You prefer to work independently. *Yes or no?*

If you answered "yes" to the majority of these questions or if you can relate to the avoidant style of being distant, consider why and how this is problematic. Any intimate or personal relationship has strong emotional features, which are a valuable asset in your life. The sense of emptiness, insecurity, self-doubt, and shame originate from our own lack of emotional connection. These issues can be overcome with conscious effort.

ANXIOUS (OVERWHELMED AND OVERWHELMING) STYLE OF ATTACHMENT

Many times, this style of attachment is called the "helicopter" mother. This mother is very attached, responsible, emotionally present but is also unconsciously fearful, suspicious, and scared of life. She is the mom who read twelve books about how to raise a son during her pregnancy. There is a chronic unacknowledged cloud of fear surrounding her everyday activities. Her frantic energy is palpable with everyone and everything in her life. Daily events and minor problems can unnecessarily escalate to a catastrophic level. She is unable to productively contain her anxiety, which spills onto the young child. The relationship bond is wrapped in a blanket of fear that is designed to protect the child and mother.

When not feeling overwhelmed by the circumstances of her life, she is hyper-focused on every move, every developmental step and gesture that the baby makes. The child feels loved but has no personal room for exploration. This anxious mother doesn't mean to psychologically suffocate her young son with unregulated emotions. Anxiety is part and parcel to all her relationships:

professional, social, personal, romantic, and her relationship with herself. The emotional umbilical cord of the mother's worry is plugged into the formation of her son's emotional life. This son, as a teenager, feels fearful, sacred, but emotionally tentative: nothing feels secure, including mom.

Safety, responsibility, and good mothering are all features of the anxious attachment style. The motivation, intention, and driving force of this relationship is terror and constant worry. The son often develops strong avoidant tendencies to new activities, change, job transitions, new relationships, and any type of sexual intimacy. Adult sons with anxious mothers don't have a sense of calmness or peace of mind, because they were conditioned to feel a looming danger around the corner.

Avoidance, procrastination, obsessive thinking become the adult son's psychological mode of operating to *never* feel vulnerable. The anxious-attached mother avoids any and all situations that could make the child sick or expose him to anything beyond her reach. The developmental experiences of frustration, such as falling off the swing or crying, are minimized. These boys didn't learn the importance of self-soothing behaviors, such as falling back asleep at night, playing outside, climbing trees, and solo play. The protective attachment was to avoid suffering by both mom and son.

There is no decline or reduction in feeling "scared" as the young boy matures and enters adulthood.

The adult son struggles with how to form appropriate emotional distance that is neither fused and suffocating or driven by fear and terror. As result, this style of overattachment feels normal, reasonable, and appropriate to him. This might sound odd given the other unpredictable emotional types of attachment we have discussed.

The anxious connection isn't balanced or proportionally guided with love, concern, or consistency. The son feels cared for and noticed but afraid of learning about the world for himself. Mom's need to control all the variables in his life continues into adulthood. Growing up, the son is told how to feel, what to feel, and what not to feel. There is an unspoken imperative that the world isn't safe, that bad things will happen, and that mom will protect her son—forever! In adulthood, this style of relating is also called "emotional enmeshment."

The desire to be a complete mother for one's son is fundamentally appropriate and reasonable. The problem arises when a mother, lacking self-awareness about her free-flowing anxiety, continually transmits it to the son throughout his lifetime. The son grows up being warned verbally and nonverbally to be safe, careful, and stay connected to mom.

Do I Have Anxious (Overwhelming and Overwhelmed) Tendencies?

- You are uncomfortable with unfamiliar situations, change, and meeting new people. *Yes or no?*
- You often overreact to a situation or problem. *Yes or no?*
- You procrastinate when you feel anxious. *Yes or no?*
- You have been told that you are emotionally intense. *Yes or no?*
- You find it difficult not to panic when plans change. *Yes or no?*
- You don't like to do new things. *Yes or no?*
- You are a creature of habit. *Yes or no?*
- You are controlling of your relationships professionally, personally, and socially? *Yes or no?*
- You prefer not to socialize. *Yes or no?*
- You dislike being emotionally expressive or angry. *Yes or no?*
- You have been told that you have anxiety issues. *Yes or no?*

Consider these questions and the degree of anxiety that you carry around and consider to be normal. Have you always felt anxious, worried, or unable to relax? This question and the ones above all point to an anxious-attachment style of living and relating to others. Your free-flowing worry is amendable to treatment once it is fully acknowledged. You can't let go of what you don't know you are holding.

DEPRESSED (LACKING ENERGY AND FOCUS) STYLE OF ATTACHMENT

Even though your mother wasn't clinically depressed (i.e., unable to function at minimal levels daily), she seemed to have little energy, figuratively and literally. Your relationship seemed lacking to you because your mother was often lying on the couch or sleeping for days at a time, never getting dressed. Mom wasn't always distracted, yet her energy seemed to be low most of the time, and everything felt like a huge effort. You knew by age five that you couldn't depend on your mother to be your safe place, a source of comfort, or mindful of you.

Your childhood was an energy drain on your mother; she was consumed with personal struggles that consumed her emotional focus. You had a mother, but you felt lonely and were often angry about small things in order to get her attention. The adults in your life weren't paying attention to you, and you knew it. This pattern only worsened with age until you felt you were living in a hotel: no one knew much about the other people in the house.

When difficult situations or challenges arose, your mother became sad, hopeless, emotionally flat, and without expression. Young boys assume growing up that they somehow are responsible for or cause their mom's emotional disconnection and sadness. Children automatically assume that this is their fault, and this issue of personalizing everything follows them into all their adult relationships. Over time, this behavior evolves into codependency, people-pleasing, and placating others.

Unlike the previous three styles of attachment, there are long periods of time without connection, interaction, and nurturing with the depressed style. The lack of energy is misinterpreted by the child as a "me problem," not a "mom problem." The young boy exhibits low energy, lacking desire or interest in connecting with his mother. At school, this child is often viewed as angry and unable to play with others calmly. Unaddressed, these traits can become a pattern of hostile, emotionally flat, or volatile relationships for the adult son.

The attachment spectrum for the depressed style vacillates between ambivalence and anger. Anger is used to jump-start you, to arouse the energy needed to maintain meaningful connections. Anger blocks relationships, preventing meaningful connections. Anger, depression, or loneliness and feeling secure, safe, and noticed are incompatible. This attachment style impedes one's desire to spend time with friends, partners, and colleagues.

Do I Have Depressed (Lacking Energy and Focus) Tendencies?

- You feel unseen in your relationships, career, and socially. *Yes or no?*
- You lack interest and desire to connect with coworkers, friends, family, and your partner. *Yes or no?*
- You struggle with self-doubt in your job, with parenting, and in nearly every aspect of your life. *Yes or no?*
- Being complimented makes you very uncomfortable. *Yes or no?*
- You often feel unnoticed and easily forgotten. *Yes or no?*
- You have an explosive temper when frustrated or dismissed. *Yes or no?*
- Your personal preference is to remain emotionally neutral with most people. *Yes or no?*
- You tend to feel emotionally flat regarding important events, crises, and tragedies. *Yes or no?*
- You don't believe that good things will happen to you. *Yes or no?*
- You don't trust people with your intimate concerns or feelings. *Yes or no?*

The mother's depressive psychological nature breeds depression within the son. The childhood low-energy home environment and sense of hopelessness are the unspoken emotional attachments that connect you to your mother. The sense of impending doom is a very strong belief for you. The world doesn't feel safe or enjoyable; it is barely tolerable, both as a child and as an adult man. These "dark" beliefs, feelings, and emotions make it very difficult for you to form safe and secure relationships in your life. However, this is not a death sentence to your ability to attach, create, and choose a different psychological path for your emotional well-being.

Secure (Consistent) Style of Attachment

Let me start by saying that growing up with a secure attachment style is experienced by about 10 percent of children. This is something that you can nurture and foster in your personal life, your relationships, your family, and your career. Emotional stability and predictability can be traits in your masculine world regardless of your childhood deprivation and neglect. My professional experience over the years has proved repeatedly that many of the underlying attachment, intimacy, and relationship issues result from emotional neglect. The long-term impact of early psychological experiences of being unnoticed, not seen, emotionally misunderstood, never feeling safe, and unable to be a kid is significant.

Many present-day relationship issues have their beginnings in our childhoods.

My experience also has shown that the men who were most neglected as children are the most resistant to accepting and healing their childhood wounds. It's very scary and overwhelming to look at our present-day relationships and personal challenges as having their beginnings in our childhood attachment styles. Let's first describe the dynamics of the secure mother-son attachment.

The young child experienced consistency with his mom's moods, habits, routines, and physical care. The young boy is seen and noticed and held, hugged, and touched. All these early acts of kindness, concern, and care teach the young boy that he can rely and count on his mother. A sense of feeling safe, loved, and cared for is established immediately with the mother-son bond. This young boy feels important, noticed, and receives positive feedback for his smiles, cries, and movements. The other four styles gave the young boy some of these acts of love, concern, and care; the primary difference is the consistency and predictability of the mother's attention with the child, which allows him to internalize feeling safe. At the opposite end of this experience, the boy internalizes a sense of deprivation. This means that he can never get his needs met physically, emotionally, and personally. The sense of neglect evolves into a sense of emptiness, deprivation that feels like a black hole inside the adult man's heart and soul. Both of these early life experiences shape how adult men manage their money, their emotions, and ability to be generous.

The secure style of attaching isn't based on perfection. The mother-son relationship has the ability to be flexible and accepting of changes; the bond is not conditional. The mother reinforces throughout the son's childhood even-mindedness: circumstances or problems aren't going to fracture or damage their relationship. The resiliency to endure the normal ups and downs of family life, school, friends, and siblings fosters a psychological experience that the world isn't a bad place and that good things can happen to me. Finally, this son has an inherent sense of courage and competency to do things in his adult life that others would never consider. This son is an emotionally secure, caring man with the ability to understand others and himself.

Do I Have Secure (Consistent) Tendencies?

- You are able to encourage coworkers, friends, and family to excel. *Yes or no?*
- You gain emotional and psychological strength from your relationships. *Yes or no?*
- You have a wide circle of friends and colleagues. *Yes or no?*
- You are receptive to making changes professionally, personally, and relationally. *Yes or no?*
- You have a sense of purpose in your life. *Yes or no?*
- You enjoy being able to emotionally express your thoughts and feelings without fear of rejection or revenge. *Yes or no?*
- Problems, differences, and conflict resolutions are normal and understandable in your adult life. *Yes or no?*
- People ask for you for advice, career direction, and emotional support. *Yes or no?*
- You have a combination of long-term and new friendships. *Yes or no?*
- You trust your family, your colleagues, and your romantic partner. *Yes or no?*

> *Our brains are wired for connection; trauma rewires them for protection. That's why healthy relationships are difficult for wounded people.* —Ryan North

SUMMARY—TIME FOR ACTION

If you have more "yes" than "no" answers, if you want more "yes" answers, or if you want secure, stable relationships going forward, this is a time to consider how you emotionally connect and relate to the important people in your life. You can ask your close friends for feedback on how they experience you emotionally. Regardless of the degree of neglect, abuse, suffering, and trauma, these issues shaped your childhood into your present day, and you can change your attachment style. We men accept the fact that we don't live or function in a sterile psychological vacuum; a fluid, ongoing process of life is the starting point for change. Remember: nothing is forever, not even our suffering!

We have the option to develop stable, supportive, fulfilling relationships in all areas of our lives. These relationship styles, healed or unhealed, are the expression of our masculinity and who we want to be in the world. It's never too early or too late to make life-changing decisions.

The pieces of your life are not immovable cement blocks unless you choose to make them into a story of misery, regret, blame, and resentment. The biggest decision of our lives is where we decide to let go or hold on to the past. This is the ultimate determinant of your life—forgiveness or blame.

Attachment theory premise: Our healing—physically, psychologically, relationally, and personally—starts with examining our emotional attachment to ourselves!

The point is that relationships matter. The most important and primary relationship in your life will always be the one with yourself; all the other areas of your life are secondary.

The most important relationship in your life is the one with yourself!

What area of your life isn't relationship based? Our brains, emotions, bodies, and psychological processing are formed and dramatically influenced by our early life experiences.

TAKING ACTION AND FIXING THINGS

Let's start with the following action steps. This is the process of healing the young boy inside your adult body. All of these recommendations are actual actions or tasks that I have done and continue to do to stay balanced and emotionally grounded with myself, my partner, family, career, health, body, and my best internal self.

- Start a journal, listing five goals that you want to achieve now and going forward. For instance, this could be to avoid raising your voice when frustrated; to consider your responsibility and role regarding the issues in your family, childhood, and career; to look at your actions from a third-party perspective; to apologize to your coworkers; to express your uncomfortable feelings; to take someone special to you out to lunch.
- Write in your journal for ten minutes a day for the next seven days your feelings about three things: your childhood, your first love, and your ideal life in five years.
- Start a sentence with someone at least once a day with, "I feel . . ."
- Tell one person each day for the next seven days about their value and importance to you.
- Practice active listening with the two or three people closest to you. Don't think about responding or giving suggestions; just focus on their emotional content and the topic at hand.
- Write about uncomfortable patterns, behaviors, or something about yourself that you don't like and that you want to heal and change. If you can't think of anything, ask your partner or children. I guarantee they are not at a loss for things you could change and improve upon. This is a serious suggestion because our closest connections hold valuable information about our impact on their lives.

These six action steps might seem trivial, but when taken seriously, they can create insights that begin to change how you view yourself and the world around you. The literal action of writing or typing your emotions, painful feelings, and thoughts requires the interaction of both sides of your brain, which creates a sense of grounding and calmness.

CHAPTER ELEVEN

MEN, INTIMACY, AND MARRIAGE

Five Variables That Work Together

The man or woman you choose to be your partner affects everything in your life: your mental health, your peace of mind, your love inside of you, your happiness, how you get through tragedies, your successes, how your children will be raised, and much more. Choose wisely.—Unknown

Conflict cannot survive without your participation.—Dr. Wayne Dyer, psychologist and author

Son, don't marry someone you can live with; marry someone you can't live without! It's easy to get married and it's very difficult to get divorced.—Peter B. Poulter

MARRIAGE AND COMMITMENT INSIGHTS— FIVE VARIABLES TO CONSIDER

The question of marriage is something that all men and women consider at some point in their lives. I have single female clients who swear at age twenty-five that they will never get married. Then at age thirty-five, she's married, has two young children, and a third on the way. These same women echo that their husbands aren't emotionally available, have self-doubts about being fathers, are still attached to their mothers, aren't motivated in their careers, and struggle with saying "no" to people in their lives. These loving partners feel that their men have unresolved issues with either their mothers or fathers.

These issues spill into the marriage whether it's homosexual, heterosexual, or common law—this is a universal dynamic. I ask the partner if the significant other has addressed the following five variables in his life: shame, style of attachment, individuating from his family, establishing emotional boundaries (mental health), and taking responsibility for his life past, present, and future.

These five variables are part and parcel to establishing a secure, loving, and fulfilling intimate marriage, long-term romance, or any type of formal romantic commitment. The partner usually looks at me, uncertain whether he has done all of those or knows how to. I explain in the following pages how to work through all five of these important building blocks for your masculinity, mental health balance, psychological healing, and improving your overall quality of life. Finally, I explain the context of why and how our core issues get activated with our partner. *Important side note: our intimate relationship replaces our primary childhood relationship.*

INTIMATE RELATIONSHIPS REVEAL OUR TRUE SELVES—WHY THEY MATTER!

It's important that we establish why intimate romantic relationships are so important in our lives, health, masculine expression, and overall satisfaction. These experiences of loving and feeling loved create the most profound attachments, psychological bonds, and emotional connections in our lives. Consider the following reasons why your intimate relationship is different from all your other relationships.

- Unresolved trauma and our attachment issues get replayed the most in our romantic/love relationships; there's no hiding our deepest needs and wants with the person we share a pillow.
- All our wounds, unmet emotional needs, and frustrations from childhood show up in our romantic relationships. The key is to recognize repetitive themes in your relationships.
- Avoidant behaviors occur when we don't feel safe, secure, or heard.
- Either expressing our opinion or fearing being abandoned for it shows us where we need to heal and strengthen our emotional core-self.
- Our wounds, negative behaviors, and self-loathing narrative fully appear in our most intimate connection, allowing us to finally heal these destructive patterns and rebuild.
- Our intimate relationship is the only place in which we can reveal our wounded boy.
- The childhood belief that the perfect relationship will heal all our wounds and meet all our needs is a dangerous proposition. This erroneous belief

leads to major disappointments (of course) in our marriages. Heartbreak within the relationship is the starting point for our courageous journey with a partner who loves us, cares about us, and has our best interests in mind.

Three Cautionary Tales—Men and Old Emotional Challenges

The three men below are examples of how our intimate relationships are impacted by so many different variables, childhood issues, and our adult choices. Men want to have a loving, caring, understanding, forgiving, and nurturing partner. Men desire love as much as women and are the least vocal about it. Although relationship descriptions may change, a sustainable love relationship is a hallmark achievement for men since the beginning of time. Our discussion is inclusive of those who choose to marry and those who do not but want a love/romantic partner or some combination of commitment and love in their lives. The definition of the relationship is window dressing, because inside of an intimate love relationship, we are all the same. The ability to emotionally connect, communicate our thoughts and feelings, have a safe psychological place to be ourselves, be seen, be understood, and be accepted are some of the inner workings of our most important relationship second only to the one with ourselves.

Robert, age forty-four, is divorced and has been remarried for more than twelve years. He is the father of two adolescent boys, one from each marriage. Robert is a documented (through police and children protective services reports) victim of spousal abuse (verbal, emotional, and physical), a victim of fraudulent child abuse allegations, and is embroiled in an ongoing custody battle with his ex-wife. Robert is a very kind, intense, psychologically insightful, and brokenhearted man. Robert has a relationship pattern of being attracted to strong, aggressive, intelligent, highly sexual, and domineering women. Robert admits that he likes "a little crazy" in his women. Recently, Robert was rewarded, per Dependency Court (California children's court for minors), full legal and physical custody of his twelve-year-old son. The Department of Children's Services evaluated his ex-wife as psychologically unfit, emotionally unstable, and dangerous to her preteen son. The department's findings and recommendations are unprecedented. Robert knows his son needs a stable, calm, and predictable home, but he feels sad about his ex-wife's situation. Robert knows that he needs to establish better emotional boundaries for himself and emotional clarity regarding this difficult family situation.

Avery, age thirty-two, divorced and remarried two years ago. Avery recently married a woman he met though his family. Avery was first married at age twenty-four for two years. Avery's older brother was a victim of a mass shooting at a nightclub when he was twenty-six years old. Avery and his first wife divorced after the death of his brother. Avery moved back home to comfort his parents and himself. Avery has struggled with depression and despair since his brother's death. Avery and his ex-wife amicably divorced; they didn't have children or any mutual property together. Since the shooting, Avery has struggled with feeling emotionally vulnerable. He never wants to experience another loss like his brother's death ever again. Since remarrying, Avery and his new wife recently had a baby boy. Having a newborn father-son bond has helped Avery to reconnect with himself again. Avery struggles with shame and feeling like a fraud as a husband, as a father, and as his parents' only living son. Avery was supposed to be at the nightclub the night of the shooting but got delayed with his friends.

George, age fifty-seven, married to the same woman for twenty-five years. Growing up, George was a product of divorced parents during the early 1970s, when divorce wasn't as socially accepted as it is today. George hated the weekly visits with his dad because his mother became very angry and resentful about sharing custody time. George loved both of his parents and learned how to peacefully manage them. His goal as a young boy was to minimize the conflict between the houses, to make his mother happy, and to avoid letting anyone know that his parents were divorced. George was successful with all three objectives. The problem became trying to keep everyone happy and calm—an impossible task. George started drinking in high school to offset his anxiety of not being "perfect."

George made a promise to himself that he would never get divorced or put his three children through what he and his older brother went through. George remembers as a teenager that his mother viewed him like his father because of his appearance, because he was a man, and because of his interest in real estate. All three of these traits enraged his mother because they reminded her of his father. She became increasingly abusive verbally and physically. His mother would have a few drinks, start yelling at George, and eventually slap him in the face for being disrespectful. George ignored these events at home and had a full life outside of the house. As father, husband, businessman, entrepreneur, and son, George struggles with bouts of anger, emotional isolation, and resentment toward his parents and wife.

These three men have to engage their emotional tools for healing and building fulfilling relationships with their partners, children, colleagues, parents, friends, and with themselves. Your struggles are real, and insight is the key to unlocking your potential. These five pieces of your personal development blend into your masculinity and how it is expressed. Let's look at the following five important elements for our well-being, mental health, and contentment. Clearing up our past interferences (traumas) in our current relationships creates a stable platform to move forward.

> *The wise person is the person who finds what they lost in childhood and regains it.*—Jordan Peterson, psychologist and professor

STEP 1—UNPLUGGING FROM TRIGGERS

Shame is emotional cancer! Shame interferes with our ability to form trusting, loving, and fulfilling relationships. Shame is incompatible with intimacy, self-acceptance, and anything of value in your life! Oil and water don't mix nor does shame and your mental health. I discussed at length the destructive residual nature of shame and its insidious impact on your entire life in chapter 9. The seven triggers listed below are how shame walks into your life, activating your sense of powerlessness and making you feel defective, damaged, worthless, unlovable, and fraudulent. These beliefs, thoughts, and feelings listed below get reactivated throughout the course of your marriage/love relationship, career, and parenting, until you pull the plug on them.

Intimacy only flourishes in a shame-free connection between you and your partner. Consider each of the following rebuttals to your primary emotional shame triggers from the past and present day.

- *Fear of embarrassment versus the power of vulnerability*—Emotional paralysis is replaced with acceptance of our imperfections, limitations, and humanness. Releasing our need to appear perfect renders our emotional paralysis powerless. The underlying fear of feeling unlovable is shaming embarrassment. The fear of being seen as imperfect, not good enough, is a childhood wound. These wounds become our psychological belief systems as adults. Your emotional avoidance against feeling defective causes you to be secretive in your love life. The fear of being unlovable is dispelled only by embracing all of your strengths and weaknesses. The path forward is embracing our weaknesses, gifts, and challenges, which is psychological freedom.

- *Angry, hostile/aggressive, and dismissed versus taking full responsibility for your life*—Holding onto past resentments and blaming childhood injustices for your life breeds a negative self-image. Hostile reactions are expressions of your unresolved shame. Anger distorts your ability to see relationships clearly without a victim mentality. Responsibility replaces your sense of powerlessness with peace of mind. Being fully responsible for your actions dissolves your shame and provides new clarity. You are a participant in your life today, not a victim or spectator. Shame is fueled by victimhood. Your shame can't coexist with responsibility! Responsibility allows us to express our thoughts and feelings in a noncombative manner. The personal power of taking action on your own behalf provides the freedom and benefit of healing and releasing the past.

- *Imposter syndrome versus competency*—This is the most common experience of shame. Your secretive feelings, beliefs, and fears are based on your early attachment issues of not feeling good enough, incapable, and inferior. Embracing our imperfections is how our competency develops. Taking professional risks and personal challenges build a sense of capability regardless of the outcome. Courageous actions transform our sense of feeling inferior or like an imposter to feeling competent and capable. Shame can't terrorize you when you have confronted, accepted, and understood who and what you are today. Shame creates a false public persona that needs constant reassurance. Competency is a self-reliant power that is independent of others' control, opinions, or threats. You aren't controlled by the fear of being exposed; you already know your issues. Confronting our fear of inadequacy resolves our unspoken fear of being a fraud.

- *Feelings of isolation versus self-acceptance*—Self-selecting actions to maintain emotional distance from coworkers, friends, and your romantic partner are common behaviors. The fear of being seen as defective, as damaged goods, as not good enough, or as unlovable is shame's strongest deception. All these unfounded fears and beliefs can be traced back to your childhood prior to age five. The experience of feeling good about yourself was not frequent or on a regular basis. In place of learning to like and accept yourself, you filled the parental gap with a negative narrative perception about yourself. Now years later, these early beliefs unconsciously guide you in creating superficial relationships, isolating yourself, and avoiding deep emotional connections. Your internal narrative might go something like this, "How can a group of people or a lover want me when I don't like myself?" Self-acceptance is the single greatest variable in developing and maintaining secure adult relationships.

- *Suspicious of authority/lack of trust versus forgiveness of our parents*—Our foundation for trust started at home with our parents. The unpredictable, chaotic dismissal of your perceptions and opinions as a child is where trust or mistrust began. When parents validate their sons' questions, concerns, and thoughts, it builds confidence within the child. Children know when things are good, bad, or if something is wrong. Having our instincts, intuitions, and perceptions valued creates confidence, stability, and trust within us. Trusting our internal wisdom breeds competency, courage, and the ability to form secure relationships. Mistrust of ourselves and others creates a belief that we are defective and damaged—shame's best friends. The mistrust of authorities, supervisors, coaches, colleagues, clients, and our partners are all symptoms of our childhood unresolved trauma with our parents. Forgiving your parents for trying to protect you and themselves from the truth or the chaos at home is the beginning of repairing your trust. Forgiveness breeds clarity and shame breeds confusion and mistrust. No relationship can survive without your ability to extend trust to the people you interact with, work with, and live with. All fulfilling sexual and romantic relationships share a strong emotional bond of trust, safety, and security.
- *Fear of intimacy versus self-acceptance*—Shame's strongest threat within us is that our secret will be revealed, exposed, and posted all over social media. Our colleagues, friends, family, and partner will discover our unspoken liability. This entrenched liability is our core shame belief within: "I am defective, damaged goods, and unlovable." Men struggle with not being "enough" and want to marry or form intimate relationships but can't allow someone to see all of their flaws or issues. The emotional reaction is to keep our romantic partner at a distance to avoid being vulnerable or completely transparent. The beauty of embracing our wounds and issues is that we all have the same doubts and fears! Because of their competitive need to overcome this deep-seated sense of feeling inferior and defective, men resist the notion of acceptance as the key to their healing. Self-acceptance breeds secure intimate relationships. Men aren't scared of commitment; they are afraid of their shame being exposed. The irony and the deceptive nature of shame, as we discussed earlier, is that shame is powerless when exposed.
- *Fear of criticism versus emotional boundaries*—Being fearful, hypersensitive, and devastated by criticism or when someone is disappointed with us is a window into our attachment-style emotional needs. How? When our emotional needs as children weren't met or we noticed a sense of deprivation, emptiness developed within us. We naturally begin to seek ways to have our needs met via searching for compliments, making people happy, being

perfect for others, and saving or rescuing our friends. All these behaviors are purposeful for the temporary relief from feeling "needy" or emotionally desperate. Our deepest attachment wounds are never healed by fixing others in hopes that they will fix our need to feel loved (i.e., codependency). The fear of criticism or of someone rejecting us is a relentless monster that we try to avoid by being perfect—an impossible task. The chronic search to feel loved, understood, and accepted is never resolved. The unconscious seeking of validation in all our relationships is a coping mechanism that stems from our childhood emotional deficits. When our boss, partner, or friends are not happy with us, our psychological state of mind goes into panic mode. Approval seeking and all of its related behaviors begin in the mother-son relationship.

Offsetting the seven shame/trauma triggers are seven relationship building blocks to expose old emotional barriers. These elements provide the practical tools to form a secure relationship with the wisdom to manage the normal ups and downs of life. When we stop personalizing our shameful feelings, negative emotions, and dark thoughts and use our new narrative, our life is transformed.

> *The curious paradox is that when I accept myself just as I am, then I can change.*—Carl Rogers, psychologist behavioral theorist

STEP 2—HEALING OUR ATTACHMENT GAPS FROM WITHIN

The seven cycles of shame interfere, block, and derail our ability and courage to have loving, secure relationships. Gentlemen, the good news is that our self-doubts and insecurities are within our control to stop! The persistent theme of feeling unloved, like damaged goods, or not good enough began in our childhoods—not with our current partners! Again, this is not blaming nor finger-pointing at our moms or dads, but rather understanding why we are the way we are!

I know that discussing our mothers can be like walking on sacred ground and our fathers like stepping over landmines. Whatever you do with this information, I strongly recommend you look within yourself for the solutions and answers. The answers to your lifelong questions and healing process takes patience. Your recovery process and journey into developing compassionate masculinity are evolving within you. No one in your past or present holds the key to your masculinity, happiness, personal fulfillment, or life purpose—you are holding it!

It's critical to our process of becoming a mature adult and having a purposeful life journey that we don't forget that life is entirely our responsibility. Sorry for the repetition, but it is an important point for any type of personal change. Our mental health dramatically improves when we accept full and complete responsibility for the entirety of our choices, health, romance, and career.

Mental Health Facts—Secure Attachments

- Your childhood family is your starting line in life, not your finish line!
- How you felt loved and cared for as a child, teenager, and young adult is more important than how you were actually loved/nurtured!
- You had clear communication with your family that was without emotional manipulation or agenda.
- When you expressed your feelings, you were believed and supported, not gaslit (denied your reality).
- Your moods, feelings, and thoughts weren't controlled by someone else.
- You felt "safe" and understood growing up.

Four Questions—Creating Secure, Loving Relationships

1. Growing up, what was your primary attachment style with your mom? (Your first thought is your answer—intermittent, avoidant, anxious, or depressed).
2. What is your present-day emotional attitude toward women, men, and intimate relationships?
3. What influence does your mother have in your life today?
4. What is one personal issue that is a source of shame and concern for you? (For example, feeling defective in your life, your anxiety, insecurity about yourself—that you are not smart enough, you feel emasculated, you are fearful of intimacy, you lack life direction, you are passionless).

Resolving Your Intermittent Relationship Style

If your attachment style is intermittent-random, you might struggle with being consistent, keeping your word, and following through on commitments. You may experience extreme emotional highs and lows, be uncomfortable with self-discipline, have difficulty maintaining a routine, be unable to follow routines, neglect yourself in all areas of your life, have a poor diet, and be unlikely to keep in touch with your friends. All these behaviors are learned and can be amended with new behaviors that create new and positive results in your life. Secure relationships are based on consistency, not random mood swings. Consistency with yourself and friendships takes practice. Your psychological and behavioral goal is to be consistent.

Consider keeping a journal for all your commitments. This would include appointments—formal and informal—promises you make, and work projects. Make a list of people you want to follow up with socially, personally, and within your family. Set a regular time once a week to talk with your partner about your relationship and what's going on in your lives. Finally, for the next twenty-one days (starting today), find a buddy to do something with, and don't miss a single day during this activity. It can be anything—walking together, a five-minute phone call, a workout routine, reading, writing, or meditating. Create routines in your life with people at work, socially, and especially with your partner. These practices begin to form stronger emotional commitments in your life. Don't allow yourself to change plans because you suddenly don't feel like doing something or you are tired—we are all tired at times. Choose someone to make yourself accountable for this transition in your relationship style.

Resolving Your Avoidant Relationship Style

Make a list of ten things that you willfully postpone, procrastinate, and delay. Next, make an "emotional endurance" list of activities, situations, and people that make you uncomfortable. Hold yourself accountable: remove your emotional barriers that make you feel powerless and not in control. What is it that you don't like to do or talk about? Your goal is to take action and approach the uncomfortable, uneasy feelings, tense relationship issues, and unresolved concerns that you know you have to address.

Keep a journal of your new behaviors that in the past you avoided. Make a list of five things you routinely avoid and then replace each of those behaviors with appropriate behaviors. Next, confront an uncomfortable situation, circumstance, work issue, family issue, or personal habit once a day. Your goal is to be completely honest about how you consciously and unconsciously protect yourself from feeling vulnerable. Taking small, intentional steps each day will soon deactivate your emotional reflex from intimacy, personal disclosure, and expressing contrary opinions. Your journal writing will help to keep yourself from building these events up in your mind. Your goal is to approach, not avoid, your feelings or uneasy situations. Any changes in your life require you to embrace them. Change is incompatible with avoidant behaviors.

Resolving Your Anxious Relationship Style

This type of relationship style is high energy, and your emotional guard is up at all times to avoid being too vulnerable (very subjective and personal). Make a short list of five things that causes you to "live" in the future. What is your biggest fear in your intimate relationship? Write in your journal the ways in which you overwhelm yourself. You learned that life can be calm, but it is usually chaotic and needs to be managed. You avoid feeling vulnerable physically and emotionally and have no close emotional connections, which allows you to be psychologically secure with your thoughts. The absence of emotion is the challenge for this style of relating. To accept your automatic emotional wall of being withdrawn, guarded from any degree of uncertainty, requires you to go beyond your predetermined comfort zone. The paradox is that your focus on thinking about the future leaves no one directing your life in the moment. Your psychological functioning requires you to be present in order to develop a secure attachment.

How often does your mind run ahead to a situation that hasn't even happened yet? Your challenge and goal are to be present, processing the facts of the relationship instead of being emotionally defensive. Identify five situations that make you uncomfortable. Challenge your limitations, and plan to do something once a day outside of your comfort zone. Ask your partner or friend to share these experiences with you. Our childhood fears still shape our adult relationship decisions. List in your journal five fear-based beliefs and five empowering beliefs that challenge these old patterns. You can tolerate the uncomfortable feelings of emotionally moving closer to your partner and situations in your life. Avoiding your desires creates these seemingly immovable challenges. Everything in your life can be moved forward with ease and new insights from your life today.

Resolving Your Depressive Relationship

Your primary goal is to engage with people. Take the initiative and create opportunities to see your friends and to have date nights with your partner. Your strategy is to connect with all the different facets and relationships in your life to change your tendency to isolate. This style of relating is comfortable with isolating, being alone, and not having significant relationships. Having a few important relationships and relating to people more proactively is your goal.

During your formative years, secure, supportive connections were not cultivated due to the lack of energy, enthusiasm, and engagement. Write in your journal once a day about something that you did to engage with someone.

We gain energy from interacting with people, and it requires energy to do it. Your emotional energy tank tends to be low, and only you can refill it. What are some of the people, activities, events, or situations that recharge you? Your second goal is to partner with someone for a thirty-day plan for being outgoing and proactive in your relationship world. Don't limit yourself to familiar situations, anything that gets you out of your house, off your smartphone, and moving changes your habit of emotional distance and aloofness in your relationships. Extroverts and introverts find a balance between their two worlds. You can attend group functions at work, socialize with old friends, and plan things with your partner. Your goal is to be increasingly more engaged with people and your life. These small actions develop a sense of predictability and enjoyment.

These four relationship-attachment styles each have their own strengths. Your decision to develop a more secure, stable, predictable, and transparent relationship approach to your partner builds deep heartfelt intimacy with one another. *All relationships benefit from increased emotional vulnerability and engagement between partners.*

STEP 3—BECOMING YOUR OWN MAN AND LEAVING HOME

One measurement of a man's success, as traditionally defined by his peers, is leaving home and creating his own. It's important to emotionally separate from our family. The mother-son bond tends to be problematic for men to manage when creating his own life with another woman or partner. The mothers often never fully achieved their own emotional separation from their sons. Incomplete emotional separation and mental autonomy creates an overly dependent bond on the son: the fundamental definition of enmeshment.

When the son psychologically prepares to launch before or after college age (eighteen to twenty-three years old), the relationship becomes strained. Oftentimes, the son feels guilty for this natural pulling away from his mother. The guilt is so uncomfortable and mentally paralyzing that he aborts the process to keep the peace and mom's favor. This strategy kicks the mother-son can down the road, which happens to be a cul-de-sac. Avoiding, postponing, and denying our mother-son issues is a short-term solution to a long-term problem. Eventually, you and your partner will have to address the issue.

The enmeshment problem doesn't go away with age, distance, or time. Romantic relationships organically require the son to choose between his wife/partner or his mother! The power struggles between mothers-in-law and daughters-in-law are a well-documented issue and often a major cause of divorce. Gentlemen, we can't take our mothers into our marriage or romantic unions! We have to leave her at home if we are going to develop significant intimate adult relationships. This issue is why men many times are reluctant to marry, because they will have to deal with their mothers' disappointment. Men will do just about anything to pre-

> *Relationship fact: You cannot take your mother into your marriage emotionally. Adult male intimacy requires psychological separation from your mother.*

vent disappointing the important women in their life, even if that includes lying to them. Men aren't commitment-phobic; we are mother-phobic when it comes to evolving. This topic warrants its own book (refer to the excellent resources in the bibliography), as does every chapter in this book. For our discussion here, it is sufficient to say that creating and maintaining emotional distance with your mother is a key ingredient to successful, fulfilling adult relationships.

Another major problem, often the most underrated, is when the son transfers his unresolved mother issues to his wife. Read that again. Transferring your unfinished mother issues to your significant other/partner is a formula for disaster. Rather than face the rage of his mother, the son simply replaces his mother with his new partner. Initially the son feels relieved to avoid his mother's wrath. What he has created is a situation in which he is constantly placating or avoiding the two most important women in his life. The problem is that neither the mother nor the new partner is happy with this unspoken arrangement. The wife/partner unconsciously becomes the son's mother.

> *Women want an adult man, not an adult son!*

"This may sound harsh," said my new forty-eight-year-old female client (married twenty-three years) recently in couples therapy, "I don't want to be his mother anymore. It feels like I am having sex with my son and it's a complete turnoff. We have no sex life." The husband, who was sitting across from his wife, stood up and walked out of the office saying, "At least my mother was a good mother." This couple never came back to therapy after this session. This couple is a sad but powerful example of the necessity of preserving our relationships.

There are several psychological steps required to separate from your mother and form your own secure, fulfilling love relationship. Steps 4 and 5 below cover two invaluable steps (emotional boundaries and emotional sobriety), along with the process of disconnecting from your emotional enmeshment with your mother. The term *enmeshment* in this context is the lack of individual opinions, independent opinions, or personal freedom within the relationship. Enmeshment can be compared to two people glued together at the hips. Son and mother blend together in such a manner that the son hasn't learned how to psychologically function independently of his mother and be emotionally aware of his own self.

Cutting the emotional umbilical cord is a courageous but necessary step for all boys becoming adult men.

The unspoken message is that the mother takes care of the son and he must never separate or leave her. Many times, the son no longer physically lives with his mother, but he hasn't cut the "emotional umbilical cord." Until this cord is cut, the son will be unable to form long-term, secure, loving adult relationships. The emotional tie to his mother prevents him from forming any significant relationship with his romantic partner. Unplugging the emotional umbilical cord is as important and necessary as cutting it at birth: if the cord wasn't cut, the baby would die. After birth, it was no longer necessary. The same analogy holds true for the emotional umbilical cord.

The fear of upsetting mom, feeling guilty, or being cut off emotionally is an unspoken terror the son must navigate. Being able to tolerate the mother's disappointment, guilt, and sense of betrayal is possible and necessary. The truth is, she will be fine without her primary emotional support or crutch—you. Achieving your emotional independence and discovering what you like, feel, think, and enjoy doing provides emotional breathing room. These factors combine to help create and form your core self, masculinity, and your purpose in life. Learning to take responsibility for your actions and choices are the skills necessary to manage your own life.

Four Individuation Questions—Tolerating Uneasy Feelings

1. How much do you emotionally depend on your mother?
2. Does your wife/partner complain to you about your mother?
3. Can you express your own opinions and thoughts that are contrary to your partner's?
4. How do you handle conflict or disagreements?

For any degree of long-term relationship satisfaction and fulfillment, these questions are critical to your disconnecting process with an emotionally enmeshed family. No wife/partner wants to be your mother's replacement. We must resolve our emotional needs and desires independently of our intimate partner. We don't want to be "adult child" with our intimate partner. These scenarios don't turn out well.

STEP 4—EMOTIONAL BOUNDARIES: NO MORE PEOPLE-PLEASING OR PLACATING!

The world is defined by boundaries limiting what is acceptable and what is not. Men who understand their boundaries and those of others aren't the subject of sexual harassment cases or misconduct investigations. It's absolutely imperative to understand your physical, emotional, professional, and personal strengths and weaknesses—hence your boundaries.

The ability to recognize your physical and emotional limits started the day you arrived in your mother's arms. Growing up, you learned you can't hit your brother with a baseball bat, you can't bite your sister on the wrist, and you can't scream in the classroom at preschool. You became potty-trained and learned to feed yourself, bathe yourself, dress yourself, and brush your teeth, comb your hair, walk, run, and felt your own emotions. These developmental milestones helped you form your identity with your family, with your friends, and with yourself.

You learned to express your own opinions, emotions, and ideas in a safe, respectful atmosphere. The adults in your life listened to your wishes—requests for what you wanted or needed—to a greater or lesser degree. You were heard, understood, and secure in expressing yourself. This everyday process of living formed a mental differentiation (i.e., boundaries) between yourself and others. The ability to differentiate yourself from your classmates is the beginning of psychological awareness of your boundaries and other people's boundaries. When this process goes awry, the onset of male narcissism—the belief that everyone and everything is centered around you—begins.

Learning how to form childhood friendships began at home with empathy (understanding) for others. These early experiences of relating and feeling understood shaped your emotional aptitude to experience compassion (understanding yourself and others) and empathy for others. Narcissist men are developmentally blocked and unable to understand or feel for others.

As adult men, our emotional boundaries directly correlate to our emotional needs being met as a child. And if our emotions, physical body, and perceptions were misunderstood, neglected, or ignored, then our emotional stability became dysregulated and unbalanced.

The opportunity to say "no" is a childhood developmental step that it is assumed that everyone learns. Unfortunately, many are never afforded the chance to develop this necessary life skill. To compensate for our unmet emotional needs, our focus shifts from our own developmental growth to seeking the attention, support, and approval of our parents. Over the years, the behavioral pattern of unmet emotional needs creates a deep emotional deprivation within us. In order to survive, we pretend and hide our feelings of neglect.

Physical abuse, sexual abuse, emotional abuse, and neglect all compromise our sense of feeling safe in the world. Parental abuse of any type tells us that our bodies, emotions, minds, and feelings are not valuable or important. The lack of respect that the adults in our lives had for themselves taught us to not value or respect ourselves.

Fast forward into early adulthood: we either learned or didn't learn to value ourselves with positive habits, good decisions, and safe relationships.

Healthy Emotional Boundaries: What They Look Like

- You don't over- or under-share personal information.
- You don't agree or compromise yourself, your choices, or your desires to make someone else happy so that he or she will love you.
- You respect and accept "no" as an answer.
- You are able to express your thoughts, feelings, and emotions in a direct manner without mentally manipulating or gaslighting the listener.
- You pick up on social cues and act accordingly.
- You don't verbally bully or emotionally or physically violate someone's boundaries for your own purpose.
- You have a clear understanding of what you want, what you desire.
- You know how to make your own choices.

These eight characteristics of healthy emotional boundaries between yourself and your partner are an ongoing process. The emotional impact of trauma in your past is amenable to healing and establishing a stronger sense of yourself. Learning where you stop and start as a man is always expressed through your boundaries, choices, and decisions.

STEP 5—EMOTIONAL SOBRIETY: RESPONDING TO YOUR LIFE

I get asked all the time, "What's emotional sobriety?" It's the ability to have mental, psychological, and emotional clarity in your relationships. You don't overreact, lose control of your emotions, or become violent. It's the ability to respond to a situation with empathy and without panicking or catastrophizing. When people drink too much, their minds stop recording events and processing situations—hence a blackout. We do the same thing when we are emotionally triggered and slip into a fight-or-flight autonomic response. We rage, yell, scream, and say things we don't mean, and after we calm down, we have no memory of what we said.

This behavior comes from the survival part of our brain. When we slip into a fight-or-flight reaction, we are no longer cognitively processing our situation but merely reacting to past emotional wounds. A cognitive response comes from our frontal lobe, our highest brain functioning. When we function at this level of cognition, we are able to consider new ideas and options. We are in our "adult place." It's our best self and the strongest part of our mental-cognitive functioning with reason, insights, and understanding.

Second, emotional sobriety is the cognitive awareness of our psychological triggers, shame issues, and emotional "hot spots." When these particular wounds within us get pressed, emotional sobriety enables us to respond in a productive manner, rather than replaying or reacting to our past unresolved issues. Shame and a reasonable, understanding response can't coexist. Shame is a reaction without reason or new information.

> *Relationship fact:*
> *Emotional blackouts are overwhelming reactions from our past wounds that replay in the present. The key is keeping our past issues separate from our present-day issues.*

Third, emotional sobriety is the ability to think and respond in the moment without mental paralysis caused by old fears or shame. This isn't living in our "heads" or being emotionally detached from the situation, but rather remaining connected in the moment. Your mental stability and emotional balance are consistent and predictable, not controlled by moods swings. You have resolution with your past traumas and related disappointments. This allows you to respond to present-day issues without a backlog of old problems interrupting the present day.

Fourth, you have the emotional patience to pause and reset when you are upset or angry. You deliberately choose to address the issue or problem at hand and do not confuse the moment with issues from the past. Your mental clarity affords you the chance to understand the other person's position and issue without the need to control or change that person's mind. Seeing your partner's position or opinion without your need to defend, or argue, or be "right" creates a safe and secure intimate atmosphere. The sense of feeling understood and seen is powerful and breeds emotional stability in all your relationships.

SUMMARY—MEN THRIVE IN STRONG, COMMITTED, ROMANTIC RELATIONSHIPS!

The following list will help you create a successful long-term, shame-free adult intimate relationship. When these elements are functioning in your life, the ability to pick and choose a romantic partner is no longer a mystery or a guess. You have the emotional clarity, psychological insight, and maturity to create a loving, caring relationship.

- Shame isn't an active ingredient in your relationship.
- Secure attachment with yourself breeds fulfillment with your partner.
- Vulnerability is a natural by-product of a close emotional connection—it builds a secure, safe, and consistent attachment.
- You are completely responsibility for your life, decisions, and relationships!
- Taking responsibility as adult man breeds respect for yourself and with your partner.
- The key to your happiness is your responsibility.
- No one makes you feel anything that you don't choose to feel.
- You have the right to say "no" when you need to or choose to.
- You have emotional boundaries with yourself, your partner, and others.
- You are able to be physically, mentally, relationally, professionally, and psychologically balanced—emotionally sober.
- Your partner is not your emotional replacement for your mother.
- You confront your uncomfortable feelings, circumstances, and issues with your partner.
- You are transparent with yourself about your strengths and challenges.
- You have the ability and clarity to say "no" to people who will be upset with your decision.

Closing Thought

Please read (and reread) the last quote in this chapter—it's a game changer. Our lives at times are overwhelming and confusing; it can be tough to know what to do next. Raising our kids, making college choices, managing finances, maintaining relationships with our wives and friends, advancing our careers, caring for older parents, and managing mental and physical illnesses, marriage, divorce, child custody, and blended families are not straightforward situations. The answers or solutions to these life issues may seem evasive but they aren't. When in doubt, confused, scared, or angry, start by asking yourself this question as a means of gaining emotional and mental clarity in unclear moments—What's my responsibility in this situation?

This question never fails you, no matter what your answer is. Understanding your responsibility in any situation provides emotional sobriety/clarity, clear boundaries, feelings of security, the ability to unplug any shame issues, to find resolutions, and to be emotionally present for yourself and the people in your circle of life. You will minimize mistakes and missed opportunities in your life when you cultivate responsibility.

> *Everything you do is based on the choices you make. It's not your parents, your past relationships, your job, the economy, the weather, an argument, or your age that is to blame. You and only you are responsible for every decision and choice you make.*—Unknown

Part III

MASCULINITY IN THE ERA OF CANCELLATION, CONFUSION, AND CLARITY

The Healing Power of Your Four Horsemen

If man doesn't start to work on himself, then the devil will find another job for him—to seek for flaws in others.—Saint Paisios

If you take responsibility for what you are doing to yourself, how you produce your symptoms, how you produce your illness, how you produce your existence—the very moment you get in touch with yourself—growth begins, integration begins.
—Dr. Fritz Perls, founder of Gestalt therapy

CHAPTER TWELVE

HEALTHY "BALLER" MASCULINITY

Embracing Your Four Horsemen

Many people will panic to find a charger before their phone dies, but won't panic to find a plan before their dream dies.—Dr. Sarah Sarkis, clinical psychologist

Stop being the one who always makes effort. Relax and let the ship sink.—Dr. Jamie Zuckerman, clinical psychologist

Nothing will work unless you do.—Maya Angelou, poet

WE ARE ALL CONNECTED—MEN MATTER TO MEN

We have covered many important issues thus far in our discussion about you and your masculinity. We continue our deep dive into the untapped potential of your life with your romantic partner, your family (childhood and present day), your career growth (workplace connections), the brotherhood, and how to be a balanced, compassionate, mentoring guy in today's ever-changing social climate. Currently, men are being dismissed and "canceled" by a backlash of anger, resentment, and repression—not unjustified and desperately needed. The social pendulum of disdain for men has swung to the side of emasculating, neutering, and dehumanizing them as means of exacting revenge. The "sins" of our fathers in past generations have been passed along to us, causing this current social crisis. The new modern masculine model of psychologically sophisticated men breaks this cycle of male injustices and "poor behavior." The trend of this current generation of insightful men challenging the "old boys club" is the beginning of men holding men accountable. The ingrained social patterns of abusive male behavior and exploitation can be resolved by men! We are the problem and the solution.

Safety, protection, and paradigm shift can't be achieved or sustained with hatred or reverse discrimination. The brotherhood is keenly aware that many of our fellow brothers have done terrible things to women, minorities, and others in subordinate positions. Men know that the tide of change is moving things for the greater good, not for the extinction of the male gender.

> *Your trials did not come to punish you, but to awaken you!*
> —Paramahansa Yogananda

Healing starts with looking inward, accepting responsibility for our inaction, making amends with ourselves for what we allowed or took part in. The psychological process of acceptance is the beginning point for our masculine journey. Becoming a respected, high-functioning, fulfilled "baller" starts with acceptance. Nothing of lasting significance transpires, changes, or resolves in your career, health, relationship, or personal life without your emotional acceptance and responsibility in the matter.

The emotional shift to open-mindedness and mental receptiveness is the doorway to finding your purpose and turning your momentum in a positive direction. The quote above by Paramahansa Yogananda is a reminder that despair, suffering, and heartbreak are wake-up calls for our own evolution and healing.

I have in my practice young boys, teenage boys, and twentysomethings who are apologetic for being male! Our purpose in this book is to help men redirect the course of our collective journey and be the men whom we can be proud of and respect. Healthy masculinity can be any type of personal expression you choose with your four horseman within.

Masculinity process of change: Acceptance breeds forgiveness, forgiveness breeds humility, humility breeds change!

Think about this universal process of healing and moving past our self-imposed fears, wounds, resentments, and shame. Old-school masculinity—"me first," "whatever is good for me" (narcissistic behavior), "Dude-Man-Child," issues of sexual abuse, emotional misconduct, immaturity, and exploitation of others— isn't tolerated by younger men. The cancellation movement will have less traction emasculating boys, because the brotherhood is taking responsibility for us. Young men are challenging their "boys" about the "male gag order" of ignoring abuse. Confronting head-on the unchecked personal, professional, relational, and family aggressive behaviors of ourselves and our buddies is a beginning point. Men holding men accountable for their actions is ultimately what needs to happen and will happen. Awareness of our mental and psychological balance and health is a step in the right direction for reversing the tide to abolish the male voice in society. Mentoring younger men keeps older men (me included) accountable, evolving, and open-minded to the ever-changing process of living.

It's an opportunity for and the responsibility of older men to expand the brotherhood's awareness of healthy masculinity and to include younger men. This may sound abstract, but I am going to break it down, make it tangible, "hands-on," and useful. I am frequently asked questions like the one above by concerned mothers with sons of all ages: "How can I help my son to be a man?"

Concerned mother: "Dr. P., my son needs to become a good man, but how does this happen when his father is uninvolved?"

What I have realized is that the mother is also asking this question on behalf of the father. Regardless of their relationship status, mothers want involved fathers to help guide their sons into adulthood. There are exceptions and for good reason. I am talking about 95 percent of families that are married, divorced, or blended, with some combination of a father-son dynamic. Fathers and father figures have difficulty articulating the practical steps necessary for the journey toward becoming a "man's man"! Mothers, single mothers, aunts, sisters, and every other combination of women want to help, protect, and guide their boys toward healthy male role models who have a positive masculine impact. This is something we all agree on and know can happen.

> *I hope everybody could get rich and famous and have everything they ever dreamed of, so they will know that it's not the answer.*—Jim Carrey, entertainer/actor

Some of the steps toward manhood—including going to school, working, and being responsible for yourself—are valuable in the maturation process. We know that a deeper psychological process is necessary for achieving a sense of masculine contentment that goes beyond wealth, a beautiful partner, degrees, a big house, travel, and personal success. The nagging question is, what's that "something" that men crave when they have already achieved success but still feel empty and lonely? The answer to this important question is found within the framework of the man's relationship with his four horsemen. Jim Carrey's statement is sage advice about men's endless pursuit of something that they already possess within themselves. Achieving professional success is wonderful and disheartening—the issues within remain unresolved. The four horsemen become a viable option once a man reaches his early forties and checks all the boxes of masculine success but feels even emptier.

A Cautionary Tale—Finding the Cure Within

Aiden, a medical doctor in his early forties, is at the pinnacle of his medical career but feels hopeless and worthless. Debbie, his wife, feels desperate because her husband's malaise is beginning to negatively affect her young boys, ages five and three. Debbie explained that her husband recently became a partner in a large plastic surgery center on the East Coast. Her oldest son asked her why daddy is always sad and sleeps on the couch all the time. Their marriage is strained, and their only focus is on the children. Two weeks later, Debbie called late at night when she discovered that her husband was having an affair with one of his female colleagues.

Aiden explains the backstory of how he got to this crisis point. Aiden says, "I have pushed myself all through school, ignoring my unhappiness: medical school, postgraduate, being a fellow, and becoming a medical board-certified reconstructive plastic surgeon. I ignored my unhappiness, sadness, and shame, thinking that achieving these professional and monetary goals would magically fix me. In fact, I am more miserable now than I have ever been. I feel like a fool believing that my professional career would eventually fulfill me. Now I feel completely lost. The affair distracts me from feeling awful and sad. It's like a drug when I talk to her; I feel good for a few minutes. I love my wife and she has been doing all the work in our marriage and parenting."

Aiden soon realized during the course of therapy that his affair was a symptom of his unresolved issues, not the cure for them! Instead, the affair complicated his life and personal struggles. Aiden didn't make the psychological connection between his unhappiness and creating a new romantic relationship (affair) as a symptom of his malaise. Aiden viewed his wife as the problem rather than considering his role, with his emotional flatness and neglect. He struggles with imposter syndrome, trying to be perfect and pleasing his critical parents.

THE FOUR HORSEMEN—YOUR JOURNEY INTO MANHOOD

First off, the four horsemen are important elements in your life going forward. They represent the primary pieces of your personality, psychological state of mind, ability to have relationships, and experience loving others and being loved. The steps for developing your style of healthy masculine qualities begin with your self-acceptance process, learning empathic attunement skills for yourself and others, finding your self-directed plan, purpose, and goals, and choosing to believe in yourself and in something bigger than you.

Each of these pieces form the fabric of your core self. The psychological, emotional, intellectual, physical, relational, inspirational, and moral value qualities necessary for living your fullest life is your masculinity. Your masculinity is you—they are not separate or unrelated. How we manage our process of becoming a man, starting in preschool through the present day, is in our hands. At some point, as adolescents or earlier, you realized it's necessary that you take personal responsibility for yourself. This realization is a significant moment in your life journey. A male who fails to take responsibility for himself develops into an adult male commonly known as a "man-child." This isn't a term you want to describe you or to be your legacy. No woman in a long-term relationship wants a man-child; she wants a partner she can respect.

> *Your partner wants you to take responsibility for your life, which breeds respect between the two of you—this is masculinity in action.*

Mothering-type romantic relationships eventually go up in flames. One glaring problem is that your partner can't metaphorically be romantic with a child. This is a very common issue in couples counseling when the wife, girlfriend, or partner is psychologically exhausted from being the only adult in the relationship. Think about this for a moment. Are you taking responsibility for yourself in your relationship?

You want a woman/partner who respects you more than she loves you. A woman can love her partner and never respect him. If she respects him, love will follow. When in doubt, choose to be respectful of yourself and your partner, then develop that relationship strength.

What's holding you back from becoming a high-functioning man? Our traumas, abuse, emotional neglect, self-doubt, depression, sexuality issues, health problems, money issues, career choices, addiction challenges, family histories of underachieving men, fatherless sons, and many other roadblocks don't prevent us from becoming competent horsemen of our own lives. Your innate ability to know what horse to ride in a given situation or phase of life is a skill you develop and use to direct the course of your life. The horsemen metaphor exists throughout literature as a group of men bearing bad news and foretelling catastrophic events. These same horsemen can take you to places and situations that will transform your entire life and everyone connected to you. Remember, any step you take toward responsibility for your life is a beneficial step in your masculine journey.

What Are the Horsemen?

Partners in good relationships have issues at times, but they resolve the problems without resorting to these emotionally destructive behaviors. High-conflict relationships use these negative traits on a frequent basis, resulting in fractured relationships, often damaged beyond repair. Domestic violence is one of the dangerous outcomes of these four unbridled behaviors.

Our four horses are going to take you to places you could have never imagined. Our masculine journey, mental health balance, and personal satisfaction are part of the ongoing process of refining our character's positive qualities, which form and shape our lives and all that we are in the world. Resisting the temptation to use these negative, self-defeating traits—criticism of yourself and others, self-hatred/contempt, defensiveness/victim-blaming, and stone-walling/ignoring—is your personal choice and personal power.

> *The reward for our work is not what we get, but what we become!*
> —Paulo Coelho

Accepting and healing our wounds and frustrating personal blind spots prevents us from crossing the line of abuse—toward ourselves and others. Verbally spewing this poison on our family, children, colleagues, and anyone in our immediate circle of life is preventable. Later, I discuss how to repair our relationships when we react and behave aggressively toward our partners. Before we go any further, let's talk about the qualities of the horseman who rides all four of your horses.

HORSEMEN

Horsemen refer to those who are skilled, intuitively connected to the horses' emotions and moods, exceptional in managing horses, skilled in caring, understanding, and managing horses. Do you see any connections between yourself and horsemen? In the equestrian world, horsemen are critical to the horses' performance and manage their overall health and well-being. The horseman and the horse become a unit. The horse needs a fully functional, mature, emotionally balanced horseman to partner with. The definition below further explains the relationship between the horse and the horseman. It's intimate and emotional.

True horsemen learn that little things matter. That anything that matters always takes time and attention, and that every little reward and release has a far deeper meaning. True horsemen learn to trust. They learn to reach out past themselves to another creature—to reach out and feel the other creature reach back. (www.internationalhorsemanship.org, February 2019)

This definition couldn't better describe our personal transformation process of integrating our masculinity into our whole person.

Five Traits of a Successful Horseman

- *Respect* for yourself, others, and your horse
- *Learning* is ongoing and continually evolves
- *Honesty* with yourself, the horse's abilities, and your community
- *Positivity* regarding your own abilities and the horse's
- *Appreciation* of the horse's effort and skill

The five character qualities of a competent horseman are borrowed from an article by Cat Guenther (https://gohorseshow.com, May 2020). The explanation for each quality is relevant to managing our own lives with respect, continual learning, and personal growth. There is acceptance of your own abilities, not a comparison to other men or what you should be doing. This truism is applicable to horses, to you, and to anything else in your life. The horseman develops the ability to emotionally connect with the horse, receiving its feelings as valuable and important feedback. The horseman and the horse develop a secure emotional bond with each other.

The metaphor of you as the horseman of your life has endless analogies, applications, and interpretations. What's important to grasp and digest here is that you are the horseman of your life—in other words, you can be the expert on how to manage, understand, grow, and become your best self.

> *The only person you are destined to become is the person you decide to be.*—Ralph Waldo Emerson

THE FOUR HORSEMEN OF YOUR MASCULINITY

- *Compassion*—how I feel about and understand myself; self-acceptance
- *Empathy*—how I know and understand someone's life, struggles, and victories; the ability to see people as separate from you
- *Your life plan*—having direction; taking responsibility for my personal, professional, and romantic choices

- *Belief in yourself and in something bigger than you*—having a sense of competency, along with the belief that you are part of something bigger than your own life

Each of these four attributes are interrelated and connected to each other. The interplay of each quality is normal and part of your personal expression of being a man. When a man is comfortable with his masculinity, then he can embrace his femininity! There is a balance within a man of masculinity with the soft nurturing touch of femininity. Historically, the old-school model of masculinity prohibited the expression of feelings other than anger or love. The three thousand miles of emotion and feelings along this spectrum were considered "gay," unmanly, or weak—feminine. This crippling fear of being vulnerable, emotionally open, and sensitive chased men onto a street of loneliness and despair.

We now dispel the fallacy that feminine emotions are a weakness but rather view them as a strength, which provides the balance that all men need in their life. When a man is mentally secure, emotionally grounded, and comfortable with his masculinity, the ability to access his femininity is a superpower in his intimate relationship. Women/partners love when their guys have this fluid balance within themselves, and their relationships thrive.

Balanced masculinity includes balanced femininity within you!

I explain the steps to ingrain each of these four qualities, along with the influence of the feminine energy, into your life and to refine your strengths and address your self-doubts about being a man. These are the basic steps to becoming a compassionate, velvet-covered brick (i.e., strength combined with vulnerability—more on this subject later).

HOW TO BECOME COMPASSIONATE

The ability to be compassionate toward others starts with you. Accepting yourself, your childhood, your parents, your gifts, abilities, strengths, and challenges is the ongoing process of self-acceptance. Compassion begins when you start to feel less anger and frustration with the younger guy inside of you. It's impossible to be a compassionate man without extending that supportive emotion to your own life. Understanding the context of past mistakes and disappointments taught you hard life lessons and not to second-guess your choices. There are three traits that help us to accept our flaws, heal our shame triggers, and form secure emotional attachments.

Action Steps

1. Allowing yourself to be vulnerable; transparent about your feelings, thoughts, frustrations, dreams, shame issues, past mistakes, fear of the future, and your relationship status; radical, unedited honesty about your life.
2. Focusing on being less rigid and inflexible about your opinions and thoughts; choosing to be more flexible with your friends rather than always trying to be right.
3. Being honest with yourself and your therapist/mental health professional about your chaotic childhood. If you are unsure if you need a therapist to work through your trauma, go see one. You will know within two minutes that this is a good choice. Journaling, support groups, educating yourself, and attending workshops are all ways to develop compassion in your life. It's impossible to share something that you don't already possess.

HOW TO BECOME EMPATHETIC TOWARD YOURSELF AND OTHERS

Oftentimes empathy shows us our lack of self-acceptance, because we can't relate to or are critical of someone else's life and struggles. When we can't see or feel beyond our need to be needed or desire for approval, more emotional healing must be done. Second, empathy for others is a mental health check for the issues we have and haven't resolved. Our ability to feel for someone else while maintaining our emotional boundaries are features of a fully formed, self-accepting man.

Stepping into someone's shoes and not wearing them home is empathy's best trait and its strength. Emotional boundaries are imperative for allowing someone to experience their own feelings and emotions. Staying emotionally sober—responsive and maintaining boundaries—allows us to be in the moment, loving, and of service to our kids, partner, and close friends. We have the presence of mind to know what the person or situation needs at that moment. The three items below are different ways to increase your capacity for experiencing empathy for the important people in your life.

Action Steps

1. Practice asking people three questions about themselves. Do not bring the conversation back to you or how it relates to your past experiences.
2. Focus on asking your partner what he or she wants, needs, and desires to have today, this week, and in the coming month. Focus on the things that are important to him or her but seem minor to you (e.g., your partner loves

cream in coffee; his/her favorite ice cream is cherry vanilla; his/her favorite comfort food is pasta; and his/her favorite color is orange). Second, ask your partner what you can do for them when they are blue or upset. What would they like from you? These types of questions allow you to focus on someone else without losing yourself in the task.

3. What situation, event, or person in your life emotionally triggers despair or uncomfortable feelings for you? These situations can be a source of strength that you can use to help others when they are upset or feeling unbalanced. You are practicing thinking of others before considering how you might be impacted or benefit.

HOW TO CREATE MY LIFE PLAN

The idea of a short- or long-range plan for your life may seem overwhelming and beyond your day-to-day life. You are simply trying to go to school, support yourself, take care of your family, and simply survive. Making rent, paying the mortgage, building your career, marrying, having kids, moving, and keeping your house from collapsing literally and figuratively are all part of the plan. Even if you aren't consciously aware of your bigger unspoken dreams, wishes, and desires they guide us forward.

Guided visualization is a theory in psychology suggesting that when you imagine yourself doing something, accomplishing a goal, or mastering an activity, you unconsciously begin to achieve it and move toward it. This is a powerful tool and works when we take the time to think about where we want to go, what we want to do, and who we want to become.

Having a plan is an idea of what you like to do now, soon, and in the years to come. This plan can be informal (a mental plan), formal (a written plan), or whatever you want it to be. Men do better when they know where they are going in life with their partner, family, future, health, and with themselves. Everyone has something in their mind's eye that they want or how they want their life to evolve. Self-doubt and shame can stop any creative thinking due to fear of failure.

> *An idiot with a plan can beat a genius without a plan.*—Warren Buffet, entrepreneur

Action Steps

1. Write down your first recollection as a young boy of what you wanted to do or be when you grew up. There might be a theme or a thread of something

that you have been drawn toward, which is not entirely clear to you. Often our hobbies, natural talents, and personal interests—helping others, animals, drawing, video games, writing, and so many other activities—provide information about your latent desires and plans. Try to connect the dots among things that might seem unrelated but could be upon deeper examination.

2. What is your long-term dream for your life in one, three, five, ten, twenty-five, and fifty years from now? Write what comes to mind in your journal (no editing or self-doubting), answering each of these timeline questions. You might be surprised by what lies within.

3. Consider a strategy for getting from where you are today to where you want to be ultimately. For instance, I want to end up in New York City. I live in California. Now I can figure out a plan to get from Los Angeles to the Big Apple. The key is determining approximately where you want to end up and then metaphorically walking back to where you are today. This is how you create your plan and strategically make it happen. It doesn't matter what your age is or your situation in life; it's about looking forward to something you desire.

Life is 10 percent what happens to you and 90 percent how you react to it.—Charles Swindoll

BELIEVING IN YOURSELF AND SOMETHING BIGGER THAN YOU

We all struggle at some point with this malaise or emotional Achilles' heel, which slays our life plan: it is self-doubt. This emotional parasite is connected to the cancerous shame tumor of fear, feeling like a fraud, imposter syndrome, and any other negative thought about us. Self-doubt mixed with shame, as we have discussed at length, prevents us from challenging ourselves to step outside of our comfort zone. When you view your life from a broader perspective, you can sidestep mental paralysis. A wide view of life loosens the grip of doubt and incompetency.

The belief that you can accomplish your goals, live a fulfilling life, and be a great man are all humble and positive statements. Arrogance—the narcissistic attitude of being the best—isn't the answer to self-doubt, lack of confidence, and fear of failure. The answer is to develop your competency by taking deliberate actions. Second, reframe your fear of being embarrassed or humiliated into opportunities to learn from your mistakes. Failure is a shame-based belief—don't forget this point. Learning from your experiences is the way that your "best self" and four horsemen take you forward on the path of your life.

Third, your life isn't in a vacuum or an isolated island. New masculinity is about being connected to others, aware of the impact of your decisions, and knowing that you are part of a bigger life plan. This isn't about religion but about tapping into the collective wisdom of others and our larger community of men. Spirituality isn't about belief in a divine being per se; it is recognizing that our lives are part of the human race. Consciously being aware of the larger picture of life is empowering. Your life matters regardless of how small or tiny you feel in the scope of things. The duality of our circumstances—feeling important and feeling small; daily struggles and loving situations—reminds us that many options and choices are always available.

Finally, a positive outlook—a belief that things in your life work out even when it seems otherwise—is the greatest determinant to your happiness, mental health, and quality of life. Charles Swindoll's quote is one of the most accurate psychological statements about the power of a positive attitude on your life.

Action Steps

1. Write down three things that you know to be true about your life experience: things that you hold as core values and beliefs that guide you and support your dreams.
2. Write down three things that happened to you that made no sense or seemed devastating at the time. Now reconsider those three events and how everything ultimately worked out, even though it might be hard to accept.
3. Write about a near-death experience you have had or a near-miss with potentially tragic consequences. Somehow, your life was spared and saved. How did that experience change your outlook on your life?

HOW TO MANAGE YOUR FOUR HORSEMEN

Embracing our four horsemen through our process of living, we encounter many situations. Some common experiences that we encounter, resolve, or attempt to are discussed below. Our responsibility and maturation as men are strengthened by embracing these challenges with wisdom, insight, and courage. The alternative to embracing these challenges starts an unconscious downward spiral of denial, avoidance, and inflexibility.

These life events on our journeys may occur now or during the years ahead. Father Time demands our attention willingly or unwillingly. Mother Nature reminds us that we aren't the center of the universe. These naturally occurring events are part of the road we all travel. Your response to each of these events dictates your destiny and quality of life in the years to come.

Aging Issues—Accepting Impermanence versus Permeance

One of the traits of mental health is the ability to be flexible about change. Since everything in our lives is in constant motion, we do well to embrace our own changes. Men who enjoy their lives in the present moment tend to accept their aging process and make the appropriate changes with aging; for instance, regular physicals starting no later than age forty provide a baseline measurement for the years to come. In the beginning of this book, I discussed Dr. J. Mills's quote about men seeing the doctor only when their penis or arm falls off. Most cancers can be treated with excellent outcomes if diagnosed early. Heart attacks and strokes are all preventable with regular medical care. I know that many people can't afford proper medical care, but we can do a lot on our own to be active and mentally and emotionally balanced as our body chemistry changes. Aging is a gift not afforded to everyone. Having compassion for yourself breeds gratitude for your physical longevity.

Aging is a gift not afforded to everyone!

- Remember, your ego can't accept aging, but you can—your life is bigger than your vanity or ego.
- No one is beyond the hand of Father Time. You need to listen to your partner and loved ones when they insist you go to the doctor—do it! Don't argue with people who love you! In other words, don't be an idiot or a stubborn dude. Do what you can.
- You aren't invincible, so ask for help. We all need assistance at times.
- Don't isolate—isolation isn't a healthy reaction to suffering. Prolonged periods of isolation can lead to a depressive cycle, despair, and even suicide.

The Comparison Trap—Feeling Defective versus Feeling Good Enough

The damaging effects of making value judgments against yourself is soul crushing. This habit might be one of the deadliest to your core self. The negative energy that you create with this habit only reinforces the awful feelings, negative thoughts, and old, punitive messages of feeling "damaged." No one has the same life circumstances, gifts, or abilities that you do.

In order to stop comparing and devaluing yourself, focus on the four elements of being your own horseman. Take note when you begin to devalue yourself and who you allow to trigger that in you. This shame-based behavior only creates despair and hopelessness inside of you. No one benefits from devaluing one's abilities and discounting one's progress in life.

- Negative self-talk is comparing yourself to someone or something in such a way that it devalues you.
- Being honest about your abilities is not the same as having a cynical attitude about your life.
- Maintaining a positive self-narrative is one way to stop replaying your old tapes or impulsive behaviors to devalue, dismiss, or demean yourself. All these behaviors are shame driven and curable.
- Men who don't fall victim to the comparison trap tend not to panic, be anxious, or lose their perspective on their own life. Be that guy!

> *Comparison kills our purpose. Our meaning and significance cannot be found in anyone else's story.*—Co-Dependents Anonymous

Mental Health Lifestyle—Negligence and Recklessness versus Self-Empowering and Emotionally Insightful

Your mental health lifestyle includes your dental and vision health and your overall mental health functioning. Your health, excellent or not, is directly connected to your psychological mental health. Living a reckless lifestyle—smoking, vaping, or drinking on regular basis—leads to physical and psychological problems. "Social" drug use is very different from daily drug use. Don't argue for approval of your "usage"; rather, consider the mental health side effects of numbing your brain, your emotions, and your body.

Ultimately, your mental health crashes, and then the lifestyle issues of drugs, overeating, poor physical habits, and self-medicating drug use have to be addressed by you. The "partying" you did in your early twenties doesn't work as well in your forties. Our self-defeating habits negatively affect our sexual performance, emotional disposition, and ability to work.

Poor physical and mental health and good sex are incompatible. Your sexual performance and desire are connected to your mind, body, and relationship habits. The issues of depression, bipolar behavior, borderline personality disorder, eating disorder, body dysmorphia, anxiety, obsessive compulsiveness, and mental illness only worsen with age and with no treatment. Your mental stability influences everything in your life. If you feel "not right" or emotionally "off," your internal system is sending you a message.

- Chemical changes occur with aging and can cause psychological, sexual, and relationship problems. Consulting your medical doctor or mental health professional is always an excellent option.
- Mood swings are normal. The longer the duration of your moodiness can be a sign of psychological and physical distress.
- Unresolved issues from your past don't disappear or go anyway. Confront whatever you are suppressing and experience the relief of healing.
- Exercise is an excellent antidepressant. Medication for mental health issues is a wonderful opportunity to help regain your balance and clarity.

> *If you don't have to go through life alone—don't. Ask for help. Accept support. We don't get a medal for doing things the hard way.*—Sara Kuburic, millennial therapist

Marriage and Divorce—Fear of Intimacy versus Self-Acceptance

Romantic relationships, as discussed earlier, replace your emotional childhood home. Your childhood home life—whether chaotic, cold, calm, or loving—is your unconscious starting point for life with your partner. Your ability to foster a safe and secure emotional home with your partner is the work of any romantic relationship. This task often gets derailed by the unresolved issues of one or both partners, which play out in the relationship. Your ability to be vulnerable, transparent, and nonreactive is a building block for secure attachment and a stable partnership. Our partners many times become mirrors of what we don't like about ourselves. The key is to accept our weaknesses without shaming ourselves or our partners. Avoiding the deadly four horsemen in your relationship is a formula for a successful marriage/relationship. If you and your partner engage in these four toxic elements—criticism, contempt, defensiveness, and stonewalling/ignoring your partner—your relationship is fractured. The level of violence, hostility, and rage generated by these four negative traits must be evaluated by you for everyone's safety.

> *Divorce is hard, being married is hard, dating is hard, intimacy is hard, and being a man is hard. Bottom line: choose your hard!*—Unknown

Affairs usually serve two purposes in a relationship: as wake-up call to re-connect with your partner or as an exit strategy to blow up the relationship. Neither justification is acceptable. Couples counseling can revive a relation-ship if both partners are willing to forgive one another and accept respon-sibility for their roles in the issues. One partner is never to blame for all the problems in the relationship, and blaming one another makes it impossible to resolve any issues.

- Marriage and romantic relationships are valuable for your quality of life.
- Having children is a lifetime commitment—think about who your coparent will be before conception.
- Your level of comfort with intimacy is directly related to your level of self-acceptance of your strengths and personal issues.
- Leave your mother out of your marriage/romance—she belongs in her own home, not yours.
- Any relationship issue can be resolved or managed if you both choose. Di-vorce is difficult but abuse is unacceptable.
- A good sex life starts with good communication with your partner.
- Being verbally aggressive toward your partner ultimately crushes the re-lationship's emotional bond of safety beyond repair or healing. Abuse de-stroys relationships.
- There is no shame in remaining in a relationship and attempting to heal and rebuild.

> Couples in healthy relationships also argue, have different opinions, feel frustrated, insecure, and bored at times. Healthy doesn't mean perfect. What makes a relationship perfect is how you choose to move through challenges together.—Dr. Jonathan Gottman, rela-tionship expert

Addictions—Shame's Cycle of Secrecy Breeds Addiction

The emotional energy expended in keeping addictions hidden is astounding. Your secret will never be as upsetting as your internal shame monster raging at you for what you are doing. The relief is only temporary while you engage in the compulsion. Over time, the numbing and fear of feeling your feelings will run out of road. Many times, this can happen in your career, but there are limits for all addictions, whether the addiction is exercise, video games, pornography, sex, adrenaline, gambling, or making money. The power of addictive behaviors is the unspoken belief that you can't handle, manage, or resolve what happened to you.

This might seem simplistic, but it is the starting point for the treatment of all addictions. You know the answers to any questions that you may have about why and how you do what you do: dive deep into your inner "man cave" and find out what you are covering up. Peace of mind can never be achieved by avoiding our deepest fears and issues from the past. The only pathway to healing requires us to expose old issues, releasing the fear surrounding them. Addictions can't survive exposure. You will replace these behaviors with actions and with people who enhance your life inside and out. No addiction is worse than any other. Stopping the slow destruction of your life will jump-start your career and relationships.

- Shame fuels all addictions. Eliminate your shame narrative, and your addictive behavior will be less consuming.
- All addictive behaviors start with a belief that your emotional trauma is untouchable. This isn't true and it's all within arm's reach of healing.
- Being addicted to socially acceptable behaviors is problematic. Work, retail therapy, heavy drinking, compulsive exercise, and social obsessions are emotional issues that at some point in your life must be addressed.
- Secrets are the monsters of our mind, the paper dragons that keep us paralyzed. Confronting your biggest secret is personal freedom.

> *The curious paradox is that when I accept myself just as I am, then I can change.*—Carl Rogers, psychologist

Loss and Death—Despair versus Hope

I hope that when a significant loss happens in your life, you don't withdraw. Being alone during a crisis isn't good for your mental health. Grief affects our brain, our emotions, our body chemistry, our sleep, our lives, and our rational thinking. Isolating often intensifies the feelings of loss, despair, and hopelessness. Eventually we all literally sit with our losses. Processing the death and isolating are not the same issue. Deliberately pulling away from your support network is an emotional reflex to feeling overwhelmed. Grief has no regard for time, person, or place—it demands our attention. Your process of grieving is solely your own and not subject to anyone's opinion. The cycles of loss are complex and unpredictable. Men can be transformed by feeling their losses; the pent-up emotions finally release like water shooting out of a fire hydrant.

Crying and sobbing are healthy reactions and productive for your mental health stability. Don't apologize for crying; it's part and parcel to becoming soulful and emotionally integrated. "Men don't cry" is a shaming myth and an example of old-school "dude" masculinity. Men cry!

Feelings of shock, denial, anger, sadness, and resolution may happen within five minutes of each other. Grieving isn't a linear process or a measurable event. There is no wrong way to grieve or to make sense of your emotions and thoughts. A major loss to you doesn't have to be validated by others. It's your loss and valuable to your heart and soul. Grief is an opportunity to learn new things about yourself, to change, and to let go of old emotional baggage.

Finally, people frequently feel so despondent that they consider killing themselves. Psychologically, it's the urge to kill off the painfully intense emotions of despair and emptiness. Guys, don't slip into the rut of despair, thinking your life is over, hopeless, or pointless. Suicide is an act based on a distorted view of yourself and a perceived crisis. This is one of the reasons that isolation is so dangerous when initially grieving and emotionally adjusting to a loss.

- Accepting the magnitude of your loss is the pathway to healing. Denial and avoiding the loss only prolong your suffering.
- Grief is a tool to manage your psychological process with empathy and understanding for yourself and others.
- Many times, the feelings of loss are so painful that you think you will die. The feelings will pass, and the pain is a reflection of your connection to the person or situation. That connection is timeless.
- Isolating and shaming yourself for being emotional is counterproductive to grieving, being vulnerable with others, and expressing your feelings, thoughts, and opinion.

Your pain is the breaking of the shell that encloses your understanding.—Khalil Gibran, poet

Disappointment and the Illusion of Failure—Victimhood versus Courageous Action

Embracing the disappointments of our life lessons is critical for how our lives evolve. It's your choice to view disappointment, missed opportunities, or failures as valuable life experiences. We know in psychology that one man's failure is another man's success. The slippery slope of self-pity, resentment, and pessimism is an issue of maturity, horsemanship, and compassion. This fork in the road of life—feeling like a failure—might be the most important. How we interpret our disappointments, betrayals, rejections, terminations, foreclosures, bankruptcies, divorce, deaths of loved ones, accidents, medical issues, and our own personal crises shape our destiny. How you interpret these experiences as a mature, mentally stable man is the doorway through which your life will pass. I can't emphasis enough how your inner critic and personal narrative of masculinity are formed by your management of your disappointments and feelings of devastation.

Experience teaches us that inside of every seemingly dead-end situation and disappointment, there are always other options to consider. The problem is when we personalize the situation as a reflection of not being good enough, defective, or unlucky. These feelings have nothing to do with the situation; they are preexisting self-doubts. Gaining our self-worth from achievements, success, and accolades is fine when they reinforce your core value of being good enough. However, outside achievements can't replace our need to grow our own sense of value and purpose.

Our resiliency to overcome emotional, relational, personal, financial, and professional setbacks is directly correlated to our compassion, or self-worth, within us. The more developed our core sense of self-acceptance, the less we personalize disappointing events. The internal belief that everything ultimately works out is an acquired skill we learn handling the affairs of our life.

The emotional quality of hope is another form of empathy for yourself. Hope views any situation through the perspective that there isn't failure, only life lessons. Our responsibility is to learn the lesson, or it continues repeating until we do. This is a tough pill to swallow but, nonetheless, a necessary one. Your quality of life, leadership ability, and life plan are all interconnected with the positive perspective of life you carry within you. Cynicism and pessimism are forms of male depression and unresolved trauma.

> *Falling down is not a failure. Failure comes when you stay where you have fallen.*—Socrates

SUMMARY

You have sole possession of the four keys of your life. It's your privilege and opportunity to continue discovering your masculinity, creating your life (rather than re-creating your parents' life), and having the courage and wisdom to do it. You will handle the journey ahead as you focus on becoming the man you have always wanted to be professionally, socially, physically, financially, and romantically. The setbacks you encounter aren't deal-breakers or a reason to quit trying or to become resentful.

Finally, it takes commitment to work on yourself, reading through this book, page by page, and pondering these soul-searching ideas. Keep up the good work, because you are changing the male legacy in your family with balanced masculinity and the positive traits that accompany manhood.

> *Out of suffering have emerged the strongest souls: The most massive characters are seared with scars.* —Khalil Gibran, poet

CHAPTER THIRTEEN

MASCULINITY AND MENTAL HEALTH

Same Coin but Different Sides

When you lose touch with your inner stillness, you lose touch with yourself. When you lose touch with yourself, you lose yourself in the world.—Eckart Tolle

The challenges you face introduce you to your strengths.—Epictetus

The degree to which a person can grow is directly proportional to the amount of truth they can accept about themselves without running away.—psychological premise for healing

MACHISMO—A UNIVERSAL CHALLENGE

My colleague, Paola A. Rodriguez, a Latina sex and relationship therapist, recently wrote an incredible article about the machismo masculine model in the Latin culture. She says the following:

> Machismo is about dominance and rigid expectations that are different depending on gender. In some Latino families, the mother begins to instill the dominance since a very young age. The boys are to be "served" by their sisters, they are not expected to do "womanly" things and when it comes to emotions, they are not given any context, and instead, it is expected for the woman to do what is "right," so their ego stays protected.[1]

This description by Rodriguez is chilling, poignant, and a common family dynamic across all cultures and countries. The longstanding favoritism of boys has exempted adult men from responsibility for their feelings and bad behaviors. Men who identify with a "machismo" persona are facing enormous pushback from women for this archaic masculine model.

The most pressing challenge facing the emotionally immature or undeveloped "dude" is learning a new way of being a man, hence the rise in a compassionate type of masculinity. The crisis of male immaturity occurs across all walks of life. Men know this and saw their fathers sidestep many of the issues that younger men are now facing. The most pressing issue has been how to be a man.

Sounds easy and complicated at the same time. Young men want answers and women want change. This is a great time for men collectively and personally shifting from the old-school "immature-machismo" man to the new school of "compassionate mentor" model for men. Mature, balanced masculinity has no regard for sexual orientation; it values how you live, treat people, and connect with yourself and others.

We have discussed up to this point many of the qualities required to grow into adulthood with a positive masculine mental health model. The new model is learning how to be emotionally expressive, relationally giving, professionally supportive of others, personally responsible, and transparent with male friends. The four horsemen give us the psychological tools for the new era of becoming a man. The guesswork is over! It is now time for taking action and applying the tools we have—no more excuses. Men love to fix things, people, and situations—this a major remodeling project from the inside out.

For instance, the ability to express empathy for yourself and others is a strong emotional bonding experience. Allowing ourselves to be vulnerable and transparent with another man is life changing. Identifying with someone's pain and circumstances is empowering for both people. Feeling seen, understood, and not alone is what all men crave. Men who experience emotional empowerment rather than hiding a fragile male ego are becoming more and more accepted by the brotherhood. Men being protectors, providers, leaders, and givers who are emotionally fluent, productive, supportive of their partners and children are vital to the paradigm shift from immature masculinity to high-functioning, compassionate, mentoring men. Young men, middle-aged guys, and older men who express their individual brand of manhood are part of the beauty of life.

Male favoritism is an issue that only men can resolve. It is no longer being tolerated by women. Equality is the new standard for men.

Machismo isn't unique to the Latin community; it cuts across cultures, corporations, institutions, and any type of male organization. Male favoritism has no regard for zip codes, countries, wealth, and family history; it is present in all types of family settings and cultural combinations.

TYPES OF MEN AND MASCULINITY

Dr. Carl Yung, a pioneer in the development of psychology in the twentieth century, proposed that archetypal male personalities exist within all cultures. For instance, the machismo masculinity style is present in some permutation throughout the global brotherhood.

Archetype is a range of basic human behaviors, attitudes, personalities, desires, talents, strengths, and weakness. Dr. Yung believed that these ingrained cultural behaviors, beliefs, personalities are handed down from generation to generation for both women and men. These particular qualities manifest in unique personality expressions, mannerisms, life goals, purposes, and motivations for men, along with certain strengths and weaknesses. Your masculinity is shaped by your particular personality type in pursuing your goals and desires and fulfilling your life's purpose.

The following list is the twelve archetype personality types that describe a wide range of behaviors, personalities, and talents. Everyone has one dominant style or type that governs your overall view of relationships, your strengths, your life motto (your guiding principle to live by), your gifts, and weaknesses.

> *Waste no more time arguing what a good man should be. Be one.*
> —Marcus Aurelius

This list is a collection of many traits, with particular personality descriptions as follows: life motto, life goal, personal strategy for achieving goals, greatest fear and strength, talents, and impact on your world and beyond.

1. *The Kind/Innocent Man—No Conflicts*
   Life motto—Free to be you, me, and whoever you like
   Life goal—Getting to paradise, avoiding hard work, being happy, being carefree, and relaxing
   Fears—Getting in trouble for doing something bad or wrong
   Strengths—Faith, positive outlook, optimism, hopefulness
   Life issue—Easily bored; life is too simple

2. *Regular Guy/Relationship Driven—Balanced*
   Life motto—Everyone is created equally: women and men
   Life goal—Form relationships, create connections; know everyone
   Fears—Missing out on life, being excluded or rejected, lacking friends
   Strengths—Grounded, salt of the earth; kind; guy next door; approachable; understanding; a good friend, accepting of differences

Life issue—Not overidentifying with relationships, avoiding his own life, finding balance within

3. *Hero/Competitive/Strong Willed—Arrogant Jock*
Life motto—Be courageous, persistent, and never quit
Life goal—Being competent by taking action; being fearless; achieving mastery
Fears—Vulnerability, being too emotional, feeling weak and helpless
Strengths—Develops competence in self and others; leadership abilities; highly responsible, accountable; warrior mentality; team player; loves physical challenges and conquering
Life issue—Finding balance between achieving and being fulfilled; not overidentifying with his body, appearance, and athletic achievements

4. *Good Guy/Nurturer—Empathic/Spiritually Insightful*
Life motto—Love your neighbor as yourself
Life goal—To help others, to protect and care for others
Fears—Being selfish, insensitive to others, ungrateful, self-absorbed, being a victim, being fooled by a partner
Strengths—Compassionate; generous; psychological vulnerability and insightful into himself and others; intuitively connected to close friends and family; self-aware; excellent colleague and business and romantic partner
Life issue—Maintaining emotional and psychological boundaries

5. *The Explorer—Independent, Autonomous*
Life motto—Don't fence me in
Life goal—To experience freedom, to live an unencumbered lifestyle without binding or long-term commitments, to explore the entire world, to experience who he is via different cultures
Fears—Never finding himself or happiness; feeling trapped
Strengths—Ambitious, being true to his soul, escaping boredom, self-sufficiency, worldliness, living a fulfilling life with purpose, ability to understand differences
Life issues—Inability to make commitments and develop long-term connections

6. *The Rebel—Aggressive, Angry, Immature*
Life motto—Rules are made to be broken
Life goal—Change, overturn, or destroy what's not working
Fears—Being ignored, powerless, ineffectual, dismissed; having to conform

Strength—Creates change, not satisfied with the status quo

Life issues—Redirecting anger to achieve productive change; finding purpose; becoming a responsible, civilized man; finding resolution without fighting; violent

7. *The Lover—Relationship Driven*

Life motto—You're the only one

Life goal—Being in relationship with intimate partner; friends, surroundings, and situations you love

Fears—Disappointing others, never feeling validated or loved

Strengths—Strong personal, professional, social, and family relationships; appreciative, gracious, passionate, and empathic to self and others

Life issues—Learning to be alone, unable to function outside an emotionally dependent relationship, enmeshment with family and world

8. *Creative/Artist/Sensitive Disposition*

Life motto—If you can imagine it, you can do it

Life goal—Creating things of enduring value, acting purposefully, fulfilling his vision

Fears—Worries about being mediocre, not impactful, or purposeful

Strengths—Strong imagination, creatively brilliant, creates a culture of insight and change, ability to actualize a vision

Life issues—Perfectionist tendencies, self-loathing (for lack of imagination), fearful of bad outcomes, overwhelmed with fear of the unknown

9. *The Happy-Go-Lucky Man—Frat Boy with Addiction Issues*

Life motto—You only live once

Life goal—To have a great time and to live in the moment with no restrictions

Fears—Boredom, leading an uneventful life, responsibilities

Strengths—Very humorous, lighthearted, fun personality; joyful with no concerns; finds the positive in any situation

Life issues—Learning to balance fun with adult life; managing the urge to escape via drugs or mind-numbing activities; embracing the seriousness of life; psychological maturity

10. *The Sage—Wise Man, Elder*

Life motto—The truth will set you free

Life goal—To use intelligence, analysis, and reason to understand the world

Fears—Overthinking, the inability to take action, lacking life experience, thinking about life rather than living

Strengths—Seeks out wisdom, others' opinions; values accurate information; shares ideas with others; understands the human process and how things operate in business and relationships; intelligent; reflects on others' opinions; capable of accepting feedback; pragmatic in problem-solving matters; not emotionally reactive in a crisis

Life issues—Emotionally paralyzed by too many options; unable to make personal decisions; thinks about life rather than living it

11. *The "Baller" Guy—Golden Touch, Gifted, Admired*
    Life motto—I make things happen
    Life goal—To make dreams come true; to understand the laws of the universe—how business works
    Fears—Negative outcomes; avoidable mistakes; being misled or manipulated
    Strengths—Innate ability to find win-win situations in all areas of life; well liked and trusted; able to develop a plan/goal and follow it to completion; charismatic personality; a leader and loyal partner
    Life issues—Lacks patience with less-talented coworkers, friends, and colleagues; being proactive and allowing others to catch up to his plans and vision; allowing others to support him; learning to be vulnerable; creating personal relationships

12. *The Boss—Leader, Man's Man*
    Life motto—Power isn't everything; it's the only thing
    Life goal—To create a safe, prosperous community, company, or business for everyone by exercising his power properly
    Fears—Being authoritarian, acting as a rigid father figure, giving control to others, expressing emotions, and sharing his prosperity
    Strengths—Takes full responsibility for decisions and their impact on others; strong decisive leader; proactive; empathic when others make mistakes; high emotional intelligence and understanding of others; fair and equitable
    Life issues—Needs to be in control all the time; unapproachable; lacks vulnerability and emotional openness; feels powerful within; lacks generosity and empathy for those who are less wealthy, gifted, or talented

WHO DO I WANT TO BE?

Personal Questions about You and Your Type of Masculinity

- What type of man are you today?
- What type of man do want to become?

- What is a "gift" or talent that you like about yourself?
- What fears do you have about yourself?
- What's your life's motto?

Masculine Applications—Male Mental Health Checkup

Each of the twelve male archetypal personalities embodies a range of talents, strengths, and weaknesses. The questions you just answered mentally or wrote down provide valuable pieces of information about you. These pieces are part of your larger persona and how you navigate the world as a man.

Oftentimes, we ignore our personal issues, wounds, fears, and resentments. These issues never go away! In order to function and survive when we were younger, we had to bury the pain and put it in a dark corner of our life. Now these issues or challenges cloud our vision of ourselves in all of our relationships. Everyone has some type of blind spot, and now we are going to address them.

> *Our wounds/trauma and fears never go away until we choose to address them. Our "dark side" is made up of the disowned pieces of our life.*

EMOTIONAL BLIND SPOTS?

Dr. Jung referred to our "dark side" as the parts of our personality that we don't like and whose existence we ignore. The unresolved, wounded, traumatized parts of your personality are as important to know as the positive side of you! What we dismiss, ignore, and deny from our unsafe childhoods becomes our "dark side." Our fears, weaknesses, and challenges prompt us to consciously manage these parts of our personality: the positive and the uncomfortable!

Your four horsemen equip you to better understand your moods, reactions, disappointments, and everyday living. The questions above focus on the unspoken beliefs and actions that guide you. Creating, knowing, and following our life mottos, goals, strengths, and challenges balance our mental health by increasing our masculine awareness.

Increasing our personal awareness breeds humility, gratitude, and compassion for ourselves and others. Awareness enables change; without awareness there is no change, no movement forward, no peace of mind. This is fundamental to healing and feeling better about your past, present, and, hopefully, your life ahead.

"Toxic" is overused in describing relationships—problems are natural, and abuse isn't.

Overusing the term "toxic relationships" to describe all relationship issues isn't fair to couples because it offers no solutions. Disappointment, arguing, breakups, yelling, rejection, and divorce that exists within a relationship doesn't automatically imply that it or you or your partner are toxic. It's imperative to understand how your words, moods, and actions impact your partner. Empathy and toxic behaviors are incompatible.

Developing a safe, secure, and stable bond with your partner is the best way to prevent negative, destructive, or toxic actions. The only difference between good couples and depressed couples is how they handle conflict, not the absence of it. Good couples resolve their problems quickly, together, and don't allow the disagreement to fester. Depressed couples avoid, dismiss, and blame the other for not fixing the problem.

Empathy and self-loathing (toxic) behaviors are incompatible!

Each member of a couple chooses how he/she wants to be treated and how he/she treats a partner. When partners deliberately choose to be emotionally distant, defensive, punitive, or verbally aggressive, they kill off any chance for resolution. These types of self-serving actions are counterproductive to creating a stable relationship. When couples try to understand each other with respect and empathy, they create a safe emotional connection and stable relationship. Acting in a positive manner toward your partner and yourself allows for each of you to change in an environment of support. The differences provide contrast between the productive and counterproductive choices that each couple makes. The outcomes are vastly different and impact their mental health stability.

A Misdiagnosed Toxic Relationship

I recently had coffee and caught up with a younger colleague, John (thirty-three years old). I want to share some of our conversation about his relationship and breakup.

JOHN: I recently broke off my engagement with my fiancée, Natisha. We have been together for seven years and the relationship had become toxic.
ME: I am sorry to hear that. What was toxic about the two of you?
JOHN: She was very inattentive to my needs and rarely would do anything for me or the relationship.

ME: Did you guys go to couples counseling and talk about spoken and un-spoken expectations, getting married, and what you both want in the relationship?

JOHN: No, Natisha said I was too needy and it's my problem to figure it out. We both love each other and just can't be together.

Backstory: John is a psychologist in private practice. Natisha, for the past four years, has wanted John to go to individual therapy and deal with his relationship with his mother. Natisha told John she would not marry him until his mother-son relationship was resolved. John speaks to his mother twice a day and sees her every weekend, with or without Natisha. After listening another twenty minutes to John blaming the breakup on Natisha, I stopped him.

ME: John, how honest do you want me to be with you?

JOHN: Steve, don't hold back. I am very interested on your take on our relationship.

ME, LEANING FORWARD ON THE TABLE AND LOOKING JOHN IN THE EYES: John, your relationship isn't toxic or anything close to that level of abuse or despair. You refused to listen to Natisha and emotionally separate from your mother. Stop making your mom the top female in your life. You talk more to your mom than to your girlfriend. Natisha isn't wrong or being selfish. It sounds like you have to make a decision between your fiancée or your mother. That's why she broke up and gave you the ring back. I would have told her to do the same if she was my daughter. John, this is your problem to address, not Natisha's to fix!

ME: John, do you love her, respect her, and like her?

JOHN: Yes, she is my best friend, and I am devastated that she left.

ME: Go to counseling and stop blaming Natisha for your emotional immaturity. Seriously, no woman wants to marry an adult man who has mother issues and is still controlled by her. Do you blame her?

JOHN: Hmm. This is what Natisha and her therapist have been saying.

ME: John, you caused this breakup to avoid dealing with your mother. That's not toxic behavior but rather negligent behavior on your part. Don't be that guy who blames everyone else for what you don't want to do.

The uncomfortable events from our past all come home in our present-day relationships. It's inevitable. Whatever needs to be addressed is ultimately for our greater good.

Our relationships require us to confront ourselves. Not just the good, but the bad and the ugly. They force us to face everything unloved and unprocessed from our past.—Anonymous

Toxic Relationships—The Most Addictive Addictions

DAVID: Kara [his ex-girlfriend] is such a fucking liar. I know she is still seeing or in contact with her ex-boyfriend. I don't trust her at all. She tells me I am crazy. I have seen her phone [missed calls from the ex-boyfriend], text messages, and social media showing Kara's connection to him.

ME: Why are you arguing about her ex-boyfriend if you and Kara are exclusive, stable, and see each other seven days a week?

DAVID: Every time I raise the question about her ex-boyfriend, Kara starts blaming me for being rude, name-calling, and acting like a jerk. I apologize for getting angry and saying mean things about her and our relationship. I tell Kara that she has used me to get over her ex, and she just wanted to have sex and use me. She doesn't care about my feelings.

ME: You know that you are solely responsible for how you feel and react and for what you say in the heat of the moment. Being gaslit is awful and can lead to volatile, dangerous outcomes of violence and death—crimes of passion. David, why are you saying things that can't be unheard or taken back?

Backstory: David came to see me about the rage, jealousy, and resentment he was feeling concerning his volatile breakup with his girlfriend of one year. David and his ex-girlfriend, Kara, break up, sexually reconnect two weeks later, and then break up again shortly thereafter. The relationship is very chaotic and unstable for both of them.

The ongoing issue is that Kara is still in contact with her ex-boyfriend whom she broke up with one week before she started dating David. On a social media platform, David recently saw a recent picture of Kara and her ex-boyfriend together. This incident got David to come to therapy to manage his anger, resentment, and sense of rejection. David is twenty-seven years old and works as a computer software engineer. Kara, twenty-six years old, is a film editor who travels between Los Angeles and Toronto, Canada, for film projects.

DAVID: I know I should stop having any contact with Kara. I block her on every social media platform and emails but not on my phone [text messages]. I feel this crazy surge of excitement, anger, and sexual passion when we fight. I can't stop myself from being verbally mean to Kara. We only argue over text messaging and never in person. I think we would not be able to be so mean in person as we are in texts.

ME: I fully agree that you are blowing up Kara over texting. The vindictiveness, threats, and criticism of Kara is counterproductive for both of you. You both escalate to a point of being out of control and saying anything to hurt the other person. You both end up emotionally drained and feeling terrible.

DAVID: Dr. P., are sure you aren't overreacting to our text message exchanges? They are bad but not that serious.

ME: The underlying problem is the psychological, physical, and emotional addiction to the love-hate relationship cycle. This is a chemical reaction to dysfunction, toxic behavior, and losing yourself momentarily in the passion of the moment. The body craves the euphoric adrenaline rush from fighting and the emotional ups and downs. The drama and chaos are the catalysts for the emotional high. Addiction to love-hate is a couple's self-sabotaging communication pattern.

DAVID, LOOKING PUZZLED: This must be why when we start fighting, I can't stop myself from saying stuff I know isn't true and shouldn't say. I think I crossed the line a few days ago when we were arguing about using each other for sex. Kara said I was a horrible lover, then I fired back. I said I have never had sex with an "ugly girl" before you. Then we stopped texting and haven't spoken since.

ME: David, you have to step back and let the emotions between you two cool way down. This relationship appears to be damaged beyond repair. You feel Kara cheated on you or at least had contact with her ex-boyfriend and your relationship is over. You said things that are unforgivable given the current addictive-impulsive reactions. No one walks away feeling good or a winner.

Any behaviors that are punitive and demeaning are destructive to the fabric of trust between the two individuals. When we tear the emotional fabric of trust between ourselves and our partner, the damage is often unrepairable. Our self-destructive, self-defeating, and self-loathing behaviors originate in our detachment from our old issues, buried wounds, and unresolved rage.

> *An environment that is not safe to disagree is not an environment focused on growth—it's an environment focused on control.*
> —Wendi Jade

EMOTIONAL IMMATURITY

Toxic masculinity and how it operates is confusing for both men and women. The two vignettes are similar in that all parties are suffering. The reasons for their relationship issues are different and very important to remember. John is avoiding his mother-son enmeshment. David is allowing the adrenaline rush and the emotional excitement of fusing and disconnecting with his ex-girlfriend to cloud his better judgment. They break up and are verbally abusive to one another. After a few days, they cool off and reconnect via wild makeup sex. This toxic cycle of abuse is addicting. John, on the other hand, is now attending therapy and realizes that he has a responsibility, a big role in the breakup with Natisha. The stark contrast between these two relationships is why the term "toxic" is often misleading when used incorrectly.

Intimate relationships expose all the areas of our life that need to heal, change, and be resolved. Raging, anger, and aggressive reactions to our partners are emotionally damaging and can become traumatizing to both of you. These reactions aren't justified under any circumstances, and they are not normal male behaviors. These reflexive reactions come from our gaping emotional wounds and lack of integration of our four horsemen.

We have discussed twelve different types of men and their masculine strengths, goals, and challenges. None of these archetypal personalities included abusive or toxic behaviors. Being abusive, aggressive, and destructive is the dark side of any masculine type. The term "dark side" doesn't imply evil or sinister. My psychological use of the term refers to the disowned parts of our life that aren't healed yet.

Any form of self-loathing, self-hatred, and self-sabotage all come from the damaged boy inside of you. The harsh feelings, cynical beliefs, and aggressive reactions are all within you, not in your partner. You are the problem and the solution to any degree of toxicity in your life and relationships.

We are the problem and the solution to all of our challenges and issues. Our self-destructive actions and bitter feelings and beliefs come from within us, not from our partners.

Accepting and acknowledging our dark side is the first step in changing our lives. There is no change in our lives without acceptance. Male arrogance says, "I would never do what the Nazis did," or "I would never hit my wife." Meanwhile this same man is anti-Semitic and belittles other races for fun. Another father, divorced, withholds money for his daughter's college tuition because of his longstanding resentment against her mother. The following traits are the attitudes, feelings, choices, behaviors, types of communication that define male toxic behavior.

We aren't talking about your partner's role in your relationship issues. Guys frequently complain that as a culture, we are biased against men because of their behavior. I don't disagree with the social or political bias, but that's not the issue and a great distraction from the problem. The brotherhood is accountable for not holding men responsible in the past for their poor behavior. One of the goals of this book is to focus on what you can do to heal, to be a positive influence, and to support your partner and the brotherhood.

Common Traits of Male Immaturity in Relationships

- Blaming others, not taking any responsibility for the issue
- Emotional enmeshment with your mother
- Defensiveness; inability to accept feedback or understand another's perspective
- Critical of anyone who disagrees with you, views differences as a threat
- Would rather be right than save the relationship—selfish and self-absorbed
- Moody—emotionally volatile when upset, gets enraged, unable to emotionally regulate self
- Childlike when things don't go your way—rages when upset
- Perceives everything as a personal attack—no emotional insight, doesn't learn from past mistakes or experiences
- Limited emotional insight about adult relationships—rejects the normal ups and downs of life; wants everything to be easy
- Avoids personal and relational issues, hoping they go away on their own
- Lacks commitment to relationships—refuses to create safe and secure emotional bonds; unable to be "selfless"
- Threatens to break up/divorce when angry or frustrated about the relationship

> *We stopped looking for monsters under our bed when we realized that they were inside of us.*—Charles Darwin, evolutionary scientist

SUMMARY—WHO AM I BECOMING!

In the following chapters, I discuss how to resolve masculinity issues and resentments, reduce toxic behaviors, and get to the source of the problem: you! The quote by Charles Darwin is a reminder that none of us are perfect or beyond making bad decisions. Everyone has the capability to transform and become a better version of themselves. Embracing all the different facets of our emotional and psychological landscape is empowering and humbling.

Our mental health stability starts with healing and addressing our emotional scar tissue. Any significant change requires our complete acceptance—no excuses—of our behaviors and their negative impact on our partners. Any type of "petty" reaction, aggressive response, or defensiveness is a form of emotional immaturity. Over time, without deliberate action to change on our part, our adolescent reactions and attitudes will impact our intimate relationships beyond repair. Our lives can't evolve, function properly, or empower others when we avoid the issues within us that are derailing our lives.

I think this last quote is an excellent summary of your learning throughout this book.

Education isn't something you can finish.—Isaac Asimov

NOTE

1. Paola A. Rodriguez, "Machismo," Instagram, May 6, 2023.

CHAPTER FOURTEEN

MONEY, WORK, AND LOVE

Male Initiation into Adulthood

The only person you are destined to become is the person you decide to be.—Ralph Waldo Emerson

Action is the basis of success.—Chinese proverb

Competition is the law of the jungle, but cooperation is the law of civilization.—Peter Kropotkin

WHY YOUR INITIATION PROCESS MATTERS

The developmental process of going from our mother's womb into the adult world of men is unavoidable. It's going to happen, and our mothers fear it, and our fathers don't want to talk about it. The three quotes above are reminders of the ongoing journey for all men regardless of our age or place in life. *The journey never ends.* Your masculinity process isn't a destination to reach or achievement to obtain. Rather, your psychological process of awakening, becoming, and being is your masculinity. We are continuously refining, evolving, and moving our lives forward, within and without. Male initiation is a continuous process, not something that ends in your teens or twenties. This trip is called adulthood, your manhood experience, and it influences and impacts your entire life.

Robert Bly, in his famous book, *Iron John*, states that unless a boy goes through his own male initiation process, his masculinity will never fully develop or form. The result of incomplete initiation is that the boy will remain boy, an immature man-child searching for meaning and purpose from the women in his life. The lack of masculine understanding, development, and experience in this man-child's life will constantly plague him. The absence of personal development leaves him in a perpetual state of seeking his mother's approval, never leaving her side or emotional reach.

These points about becoming a man or remaining a boy are shocking, scary, and true. Your masculinity will not be found in a woman; it has to be discovered within yourself and the brotherhood. Likewise, a young woman's femininity is contained within herself and the sisterhood. Women need women as much as men need men. This a wonderful energy source for both men and women, connecting with their own people. This isn't a conflict; it's a natural developmental process.

> *Male initiation does not move toward machoism; on the contrary, it moves toward achieving a cultivated heart before we die.*
> —Robert Bly, poet, author

The dynamic of searching for masculine wisdom in a lover, girlfriend, sister, or mother is often referred to being a "mama's boy." Unfortunately, this man never feels or experiences his true core essence of being a mature, wise, masculine soul through women. It's not a woman's responsibility or burden to teach a boy about manhood. Often a mother tries because the men in her son's life are nonexistent. We love these women and their incredible effort.

The crisis point lights a fire inside of men to help younger men with the process of growing up. Men help men to become civilized, mentally balanced men. Women know that their sons, brothers, and partners need to be surrounded by responsible mentoring men. All expressions of masculinity innately lead, teach, support, and mentor young men on their journey. Sharing and paying forward to the next generation of men is an inner jewel that shines within an older man. This is an example of success and being fulfilled as a man.

Growing up is an inevitable and necessary process. Three areas on our masculine journey—money, career/work, and romantic/marriage relationships—are pressure points for us, moments of maturation at which we accept and courageously move forward with our life plans. Each of these milestones is an indicator of the quality of life we choose and desire. It's not the title or the job we do that matters as much as our emotional connection to it. The depth of fulfillment that we experience and how our life unfolds is in our hands. It's impossible to sidestep these inevitable markers along our path. Men need to reach these different milestones for the greater good of the brotherhood.

TWO BIG CHALLENGES FOR MEN: MONEY AND WORK

> *Nobody is going to pour truth into your brain. It's something you have to find out for yourself.*—Noam Chomsky

Your Masculinity and Money

The topic of money is a universal subject that men confront every day. Everyone has opinions about money, the desire for it, and motivation to earn it. In the introduction, we discussed Jeffrey Epstein's psychopathic behaviors and destructive manipulation that he camouflaged with immense wealth, power, and social status. Money can be corrupted when it is used as a tool for control, power, and self-esteem. Epstein's lack of accountability and responsibility epitomizes the dark side of money.

The brotherhood now questions the unspoken cultural male desire to be the guy who has more money than God. Wealth doesn't necessarily imply a psychologically balanced individual or a mentally healthy or empathic man. We all know this, but we sometimes seem to be blinded to this fact. Money and issues related to money are topics by which men define themselves.

Money for centuries has been used as a socially acceptable coping mechanism for a man's unresolved mental health issues. If you are

> **Money and men are no longer privileged.**

wealthy or own a business, you have been given a free pass for your inappropriate behavior by the brotherhood. It's the "guy code" for admiring one's financial prowess. Meanwhile, women are no longer tolerating wealthy, abusive men in the workplace or professional setting. Women now want the same social benefits that men have been afforded with wealth, prestige, and positions of influence.

Money isn't evil. Men make poor choices and good choices with money. Economics is a vehicle that can be used for the greater good or not. Men's obsession with wealth, status, and large sums of money can be a sign of unresolved mental health issues. Often the motivation for making money is a symptom of deeper unresolved issues, traumas, and emotional deprivation. It's our relationship with money, how we use it, and value we place on it that can be problematic or beneficial. Again, we decide how we relate to having power, using our wealth constructively or using it to control our ex-partners, our children, and the people around us.

Greed is good!—Gordon Gekko, *Wall Street*

Our psychological issues surrounding self-worth influence our relationship to money and our career choices. Earning large sums of money, accumulating wealth, and being a savage businessman is socially esteemed by other men.

The movie *Wall Street*, starring Michael Douglas and Charlie Sheen, depicts a hungry, highly motivated young stockbroker (Charlie Sheen) who is willing to do anything to get to the top of the finance world, including illegal insider trading. This crime relates to selling or buying a company's stock based on inside information, such as a company's earnings or losses, before the news is public. The profits from these activities benefit only the men involved. These behaviors, choices, and lack of empathy come from a psychological childhood attachment issue.

Money's Big Secret—Emotional Deprivation

Gordon Gekko's quote typifies the attitude that greed supersedes one's values and other people's lives and disregards the impact of these decisions. Business can be ruthless, heartless, and soulless when conducted by men psychologically unaware of the ramifications of prioritizing profits over people. The men running your company, your bank, and your retirement fund can be insightful and ethical. Money is a conduit for greed, selfishness, theft, embezzlement, fraud, and many other negative behaviors and actions, which are all motivated by emotional deprivation.

Emotional deprivation, as it applies to our discussion, is as follows: *a lack of adequate interpersonal attachments that provide affirmation, love, affection, and interest, especially on the part of the primary caregiver during a child's developmental years.*

The insatiable longing to feel loved, accepted, and understood follows you into adulthood unconsciously. Attempting to use money and all its accolades—filling the hole of deprivation within your heart and soul—leads to greed. There was never enough love and attention growing up, and there will never be enough money or enough anything. It's the psychological belief that you will never have enough, the emotional state of feeling insatiable, which makes money a dangerous companion. Greed is a natural by-product of emotional deprivation.

Childhood deprivation breeds adult greed and entitlement.

Resolving our emotional sense of feeling damaged, unlovable, not good enough, or not valuable is never accomplished from the outside. In fact, the disappointment that comes from doing great things in business and still feeling empty is traumatic. Money can't fill, heal, or adequately address the lack of emotional attention, affection, understanding, and support that we felt while growing up. Our emotional health began in our childhood and continues to this very moment. You can't hide your psychological wounds in the closet. Your emotional and mental health is as vital to your life as the health of your cardiovascular system. You can't live without either of them.

Business is necessary and productive, but it will never be a replacement or substitution for your personal healing, growth, and transformation. As we have discussed throughout the book, our early childhood issues can only be addressed from within. No amount of money can compensate for what you didn't receive as a young boy! In chapter 16, I discuss how to heal our inner young man, our adult man, and our deepest fears. Remember, greed is a belief that there isn't enough for you. Not experiencing enough emotional attention, safe connections, or affection growing up is the same despair as not making or having enough money.

Men have glorified the pursuit of money and the power it commands. Other movies such as *Wall Street: Money Never Sleeps, The Big Short,* and *The Wolf of Wall Street* depict the turbulent lives of the individuals involved in world

> *Greed always betrays and slays its followers.*

finance and their global impact. Each movie leaves the viewer with a sense of emptiness and despair when the heroes are finally taken down by their greed. The point is that your relationship with money starts with you, which directly relates to your sense of emotional fulfillment and stability.

A Cautionary Tale—Money and Feeling Defective

I was referred a client, Charles, a married thirty-one-year-old bartender who struggles with drinking and bouts of self-doubt and shame. Charles and I met for several sessions, and during one particular therapy session, Charles expressed his hopelessness about ever being self-supporting.

CHARLES: I feel terrible on the first of each month when I don't have enough money to cover my bills. I get very sad, hopeless, and feel awful. I will not hurt myself, but I feel like a loser, not having enough money for my wife and myself. Fortunately, my wife has a good job, and she handles most of the house expenses. I am paying off my graduate school loans from before our marriage [he had been married two years].

ME: What's the narrative in your head about you and money?

CHARLES: I feel that if I was "man" enough, successful enough, or getting my act together, I wouldn't have these money issues. Then I cycle into hating myself about my financial situation. My wife gets mad because she wants me to stop beating myself up.

ME: Charles, do you believe that you deserve to have a good job and fulfill your dreams of selling TV or movie scripts? You moved to Los Angeles from Wisconsin for this reason, right?

CHARLES: I think I have felt bad about myself for as long as I can remember.

ME: Charles, your issues with money might be connected to your beliefs about feeling defective, not good enough, and that you deserve to struggle.

CHARLES: *Yes!* I guess I really do feel that way and didn't see the connection between my shame and having enough.

You and Your Relationship to Money

- How does it feel or would feel if you had immense wealth?
- How important is money to your sense of self or self-image?
- What feels missing or lacking in your life that money can't buy?
- Can you be successful without making money?
- How does your money impact your masculinity?

Men, Careers, and Work

Men for centuries have been ruthlessly judged for their ability to go out into the wilderness, hunt for their family, and protect them. These basic skills factor into all the archetypes, masculinity styles, and how men continue to view themselves. Our discussion about money could be its own book and only scratch the surface of its impact on men. The other side of the money coin for men is work. Careers, work, and how you make a living are fundamental questions that all young men ask themselves and must resolve. A major pitfall that absolutely must be dispelled is the belief that certain jobs, careers, occupations are not masculine! This couldn't be any further from the truth and is major cause of distress for many young men.

Your choice of a job doesn't define your masculinity; it is only one expression of it!

Your masculinity is much bigger than your net worth, job, or the company you own or run.

Feminizing a career is a dangerous icy slope. Men's mental health is the combination of the masculine and feminine parts of you harmoniously interacting together. The exclusion of one's feminine qualities—feelings, emotions, nurturing—is detrimental to one's masculine expression and mental health stability. It's very difficult to run through life on one leg when you have the full use of another healthy leg. We need full access to our psychological and mental capacities to productively manage our lives, no more barriers or self-imposed restrictions because of a bias against the feminine resource within us.

The despair of figuring out how to support yourself and what to do with your life are universal questions that everyone faces. The uncertainty of finding a job automatically launches you into adulthood. Career questions start your journey into the hard, cold, masculine world of selling and buying business. The natural maturation process of working causes many to panic. These necessary life steps often generate old feelings of being unsupported, fatherless, directionless, and lost. Having the patience and courage to find a job/passion that you love, enjoy, and do for work is ideal. Remember that any urgency you may feel to find a job might be motivated by your unresolved sense of emotional deprivation.

Discovering your professional interests, desires, wishes, and abilities requires you to commit yourself to a career track. Narrowing down the activities and occupations that seem interesting to you can be overwhelming. The field that you work in isn't as important as your motivation to work in that particular field, whether it's medicine, finance, carpentry, automotive, real estate, accounting, public service, nonprofit, book publishing, theater, education, law, gaming, computer science, medicine, nursing, teaching, social work, food services, sports industry, fashion, mental health, and twenty-five thousand other options.

> *The urgency to figure out our career and life is immediate gratification, fueled by our fear of the unknown. Your life is a series of unknown events that become sources of comfort and peace of mind.*

It's imperative to remember that your career, job, or vocation doesn't define your masculinity; it is one expression of it. Many men, including me, have bought into this illusion of a "man's job" not including certain professions. This is a myth that impairs ambition, dreams, and finding your life's purpose.

Find a job you love, and you will never have to work a day in your life.—Confucius

The old-school business model of competitiveness and cutthroat tactics is now being questioned by women in the workplace. The increasing number of women entering the workplace in the last twenty years has helped to civilize the hunt-or-be-hunted approach to how business is conducted and people are treated in the workplace. The feminine value of relationships and integrity are being prioritized over profit margins and work first, family second business models. What you do for a living is secondary to what kind of a person you are.

Often, our lack of self-acceptance leads us to feeling defective and damaged, which inhibits our ability to maximize our career potential regardless of the profession. We could spend countless hours discussing the male culture of competition, which has many flaws and inherent abuse built into it. Suffice it to say that any degree of abuse that we engage in has to be questioned. The new masculinity of insight, awareness, and mental health balance can't turn a blind eye to this emotional cancer in men and the workplace. Men can treat men with respect without compromising their careers.

Ruthless, soulless, and destructive competitiveness isn't good business, it's uncivilized behavior for the sake of profit.

Another career myth men have bought into is that a big career will offset our inner personal issues. Wealth can't offset your personal issues, resolve your challenges, and emotionally fulfill you. Personal healing can't be brought into the workplace with the idea that your boss's or colleagues' role or responsibility to heal you. Your job or your boss isn't responsible for resolving your psychological fears by the third quarter of next year. Your job, career, profession, and occupation are pieces of the bigger picture of your life, your purpose, and your fulfillment. The hub of your life is you, not what you do or the money you make. Those parts are pieces of your life's fabric. Mental health balance is interacting with all the different parts of your life with a sense of equality and purpose.

The beliefs underpinning ageism—prejudice or discrimination based solely on age, not on ability, experience, or capacity—are a myth. Culturally, men have been programed with the idea that by certain age, you will have (or should have) accomplished certain things.

You don't reach your work/career potential until your sixties, and it continues into your eighties. Read this again.

Otherwise, you missed the boat and failed (feelings of shame). This is an illusion based on emotional deprivation. If you don't reach your career goals by age thirty-two, you are not missing your own parade. Your parade hasn't even started. The maturation process isn't a straight line or a smooth road. The fear of not making things happen quickly enough or reaching imaginary markers of success is an old issue. Remember, anxiety lies—everything isn't urgent or a crisis.

Emotional Deprivation Increases Feelings of Shame in the Workplace

Our feelings of emptiness (emotional deprivation) will always lie to you and tell you that you are inadequate and lack the skills necessary to move forward. Our free-flowing feelings of shame blend into our inner sense of emotional despair and self-loathing. The myth that we could find fulfillment if only we did something better, were smarter, taller, more popular, went to a better school, trained better, or were better connected is self-defeating. Shame and its friends distort your ability to see yourself and others objectively. Notice that each bullet point below starts with "you." The unspoken belief that you will never succeed or get where you want to go are illusions, old wounds that are not relevant today. The idea that you are defective is an old issue with a new face: your career and work life. Shame and self-doubt create our inner narrative, such as:

- You are too slow.
- You are not growing quick enough.
- You aren't making enough money.
- You are falling behind your peer group.
- You aren't good enough; everyone is better.
- You are unlikable and unpopular.
- You are . . .

Professional clarity—or for that matter any type of clarity—requires honesty and vulnerability. Our past fears aren't our current work problems. The alternative is mental and emotional confusion of repeatedly reliving your past in the present moment. The challenge is keeping those unprocessed traumas from clouding our current work life and not allowing the two to mix.

Mental health professionals encourage you to have goals. Because you haven't reached a particular position or career doesn't necessarily negate the value of your current job. The life experience and lessons you learn now will benefit you many years later. Impatience with yourself or the job often covers up unresolved emotional disappointments. The panic of never reaching your goal, accomplishing what you want, or getting where you want to go is another form of emotional deprivation. The uneasy, *dis*ease feelings that you will not get what you want now or in the future are a source of chronic anxiety and fear. The ability to trust in yourself and be patient with your career process is indicative of a secure emotional attachment to yourself and your internal world.

Know Your Purpose

Each decade of your life holds a certain career purpose, objectives, and necessary experiences. Accept that your masculine journey is planning

Adult clarity requires separating your past fears from your current frustrations—not blending them together.

for the long game, not immediate flash-in-the-pan success. Consider the following building blocks of personal success, finding your purpose, and creating a positive career path.

- Twenties—Gain a variety of different work experiences by trying different jobs to find out what you like and don't like. Gaining work experience is the goal; nothing is binding or lifelong unless you decide.
- Thirties—Focus on a field or profession; choose a path to start building your career foundation; make a conscious commitment to a career direction. You choose the direction of your career while keeping an open mind about adjusting it as you go.
- Forties and fifties—Master your craft: become an expert with more than ten thousand hours of experience doing it. This twenty-year phase is the middle of your career cycle; plant seeds for your future and develop your expertise.
- Sixties through eighties—Maximize your years of productivity, potential, and expertise. You have achieved the highest levels of productivity and experience. This period in your life, whether active, semi-active, or retired, is a result of your persistence throughout your work life.

A study published in the *New England Journal of Medicine* (6/2018) found that people reach their peak career potential at age sixty, and this trend continues into their eighties. The study reports that between the ages of sixty to seventy and seventy to eighty represent the best and second-best levels of a person's professional work life. This study is consistent with developmental psychology theories that suggest that with aging comes expertise to mentor, teach, and lead others. These types of activities breed fulfillment, contentment, and generosity. *This is our career goal: empowering others and sharing years of knowledge with younger men and women.* There are many things that money can buy, but one thing it can't buy is professional experience—it's priceless!

Doubt kills more dreams than failure ever will.—Suzy Kassem

Your job search, career path, and professional development isn't a time-limited endeavor; it's a lifetime project. The self-induced panic that your career isn't progressing fast enough is a distraction from your personal growth and life plan. Finding a job that "works" for your lifestyle, family situation, and mental health is a process that takes time and many twists and turns. Ultimately, it's possible to be where you need to be and whom you choose to be: this is one of many ways your balanced, healthy masculinity expresses itself.

Finally, your work ethic is a reflection of your psychological commitment to your life plan, goals, and hopes. Each generation criticizes the younger generation for being lackadaisical about work and expecting a "free ride." People who are motivated, personally driven self-starters have a clear idea of what they want, what their goal is, and where they are going. These traits are not age dependent but are focus driven.

What's My Work Ethic

Your work ethic is a window into your psychological connection to yourself. Your maturity breeds the courage within to overcome self-doubt. Your short-term and long-term plans maintain a healthy balance between courage and fear. The quote above is the foundation of your career launching point. Self-doubt results in failure to launch. The lack of planning, unclear purpose, and not spending the time to truly figure out your next step injects fear and self-doubt into you. Your work and life plan automatically builds confidence and competency to pursue what is unseen, launching you in that direction. Concerns about career direction, work ethic, and motivation are nonissues when you engage and embrace your life plan.

You are responsible only for taking the next step, knowing that it will get you where you ultimately want to be. Work pressure, money concerns, and feeling secure on your career path

Remember, overnight success takes fifteen years!

with economic uncertainty are part and parcel to the world of business. Your inner rock of confidence keeps you from riding the highs and lows of the latest news on Wall Street. Keeping a positive attitude when things feel shaky is one of your superpowers of your masculine journey.

Questions about Career Goals and Purpose

- If you could do anything for work, what would it be?
- Do you have difficulty making choices? If so, why?
- What is something that makes you feel loved and secure?
- When you feel emotionally insecure, how do you compensate for it?
- How important is social status in your job selection?
- What are some of your strengths?
- What is an area or issue in your life that could be a detriment to your career growth, and what are you doing about it?
- What is your long-term career goal?

Stand true to your calling to be a man. Real women will always be relieved and grateful when men are willing to be men.
—Elisabeth Paglia

SUMMARY—BUILDING YOUR MASCULINE FOUNDATION

The value of balanced masculinity is balanced mental health.

- Compassion: Being vulnerable in your professional life
- Empathy: Resolving shame, which distorts your beliefs about yourself and others
- Life plan: Setting goals for following your passions and interests
- Belief in yourself and something bigger than you: Recognizing that your life impacts more than just yourself
- Ability to navigate your challenges, disappointments, accomplishments, and build secure relationships: Managing each of these areas of your life in a productive manner for yourself and your partner and family

Each of these aspects of your life are major influences and cornerstones in your career, partner selection, and relationship with money. Having empathy for yourself and others prevents the development of any type of abusive, destructive, or toxic behavior in your relationships. The things you truly want start with feeling fulfilled within yourself. We have covered a tremendous amount of territory that all men face along their masculine journey. Each element is as valuable as the other and requires your full attention to manage it.

Most people are searching for happiness outside of themselves. That's a fundamental mistake. Happiness is something you are, and it comes from the way you think.—Wayne Dyer, author

CHAPTER FIFTEEN

THE MAKING OF A MAN

Balanced Masculinity

Genius is the power of carrying the feelings of manhood into the powers of manhood.—Samuel Taylor Coleridge

A real man loves his wife and places his family as the most important thing in life. Nothing has brought me more peace and contentment in life than simply being a good husband and father.—Frank Abagnale

The only person you are destined to become is the person you decide to be.—Ralph Waldo Emerson

A CAUTIONARY TALE—"WORK WAS MY IDENTITY"

Matt is a forty-six-year-old married father. Matt was referred to me by his medical doctor for chronic anxiety and obsessive-compulsive behaviors. Matt lost his job three months earlier and hasn't felt "normal" since then. He immediately began checking his bank account balances and stocks every ten minutes all day long to reassure himself that he wouldn't become homeless. The conversation below illustrates Matt's psychological confusion, sense of betrayal, resentment, loss of identity, and feelings of no longer belonging.

MATT: I was laid off, forced retirement, or whatever they call it for getting rid of the highest earners in the company. The new CEO is a prick and someone I have known for fifteen years. He used to work for me when he first came to the company fifteen years ago. He is a mercenary whose only goal is bottom-line profit. My real estate team had several older men (fifty-five years and older) with twenty-plus years with the company, whom he forced out in the fourth quarter of last year. I was told at that time that my team— department for commercial real estate investments—was not in jeopardy of being disbanded. I was wrong. I don't want to hate him [boss] or the executive board, but I am very upset. My whole life seems like a waste now.

ME: Why do you think and feel your life is over and everything is ruined?

MATT: I have lost my identity, losing this job. I know it sounds bad but that's how I feel. I lost my professional relationships, close friendships on our team, and social prestige I felt. Now I am that guy who calls my friends to meet for lunch and they are unable to for six weeks. I feel like a loser.

ME: What are you doing during the day now that you aren't going to work?

MATT: I can't get myself motivated to get off the couch and go to the gym, reach out to other colleagues, network, or even go for walks with my wife. I literally sit on the couch for three, four hours at a time staring at the wall.

Backstory: Matt was in his late teens when his father made some poor business decisions and lost his four car dealerships in California. The financial losses caused his father to declare bankruptcy. After the family's financial crisis, his father never seemed to be the same. The loss of his job triggered Matt's repressed memories about his father's depression and fear of losing everything. The irony is that Matt has a significant economic cushion valued at more than $15 million and has professional options. His father's sadness has never left his mind or heart.

ME: Matt, do you think there is any connection between your job loss and your father's financial crash? Maybe there are some underlying emotional connections between you and your father? The trauma of watching your father lose everything and losing your job has to be emotionally overwhelming.

MATT: I know I have been pushing myself since the crisis to not end up like my father, a broken man. My father came to this country in the early 1960s and worked his way up in the automotive business. My dad had no money or family support when he came here from Europe. I have always been proud of him. My wife says I place too much importance on my career and making money.

If trauma can be passed down through generations, then so can healing!

Matt's story isn't unusual for men overcompensating in their careers to offset their emotional traumas. How do we men appropriately develop outlets for our emotional fears and worries about money without losing our souls?

The answer begins with building your core sense of self, which is untouchable by the outside world. The tools necessary for developing your core self start with your self-acceptance dynamics, which continually evolve throughout your life. Your core foundation blends together and connects all the different facets of you—emotional cohesiveness. These bonds form your personal beliefs, direct your psychological functioning, impact your physical health, facilitate your relationship style, your life plans, and your desires. Nothing in your life functions without going through your core self; it's the center of your life.

Let's take a look at the steps necessary to build, rebuild, strengthen, and continue building you. This may sound like Build-a-Bear Workshop, which it is and isn't. You have the agency to choose, amend, rewrite, reprogram, expand, delete, heal, and create the type of man you want to be. The Build-a-Bear store offers so many options for kids to choose the kind of bear they want to create. The analogy holds true for us. Men love to fix and build things! So let's enlist the brotherhood to build masculine men who can help heal the brothers stranded on the side of the road in their life.

BUILDING YOUR LIFE FROM
THE INSIDE—YOUR DESIGN PROJECT

Self-love, self-respect, self-worth. There is a reason they all start with "self." You cannot find them in anyone else.—Ram Dass

Frequently, my clients ask me the following types of questions: "How do I get rid of my self-doubts"; "How can I feel better about myself"; and "How do I stop caring about what other people think of me?" These questions and ones like them all come from the same place inside of us—our core self. I have referred to your sense of self as your "gold brick," which shame covers with mud, fear, and despair. Our self-acceptance, self-worth, and self-respect all originate from within you—the core you! I explain to my clients that they have an inner self that needs to be developed, strengthened, understood, and engaged. At this point, they stare at me like my dog does, with a blank look of incomprehension.

We discuss the process in terms of self-growth and different applications for building the man within you. The idea that we can be the author of our own story provides a sense of hope. Please reread the three quotes at the start of the chapter. Each one is a poignant reminder of the importance of embracing our manhood.

For clarification purposes, let's differentiate among three important components of you:

- core self
- self-acceptance
- separation/individuation

Each component has its own dynamic: simultaneously interrelated and separate from the others. Confusing? Be patient and this will come together as we bring the pieces of your life into focus. You are going to connect the dots about yourself that have been question marks for years. The unseen links between your moods, personality disposition, relationship patterns, career opportunities, and luck in life aren't random.

THREE COMPONENTS OF YOUR FOUNDATION

Definition of Your Core-Self

Your core self is the command center of your being, feelings, and psychological functioning. It's the hub of your moral and emotional ideas and beliefs that consciously and unconsciously direct your choices. The statement, "I believe in my core that . . ." is an example of your intuitive gut feelings, your core self that guides you in your choices, your inner voice of reason and what's important to you. Every part of your life is connected to your core self: your body, your health choices, partner choices, sexual choices, career path, emotions/feelings, your money choices, your perspective on life, and your moral compass. This is the unmovable foundation within you that everything else comes from.

Mental health and mental illness start with your ability to be psychologically integrated with your life or detached from it.

As an adult, your challenge is to reconnect with your inner self and wipe off all the mud (shame) that blocks you from you. We have discussed our shame factor, and you have the tools to disconnect your shame triggers and understand the scared, lonely young boy inside of you.

Whatever you do requires you to connect with your core self. This connection becomes your internal guide, and without it you are detached from yourself and your destiny. Men who are lost professionally and lack a plan and focus are disconnected from their inner selves. You can't live on the outside and think that it will satisfy the inside parts of yourself.

Unhappy men have one thing in common: a wounded boy inside of them screaming for attention and help.

Read that again!

You can't be guided by your values, morals, and mental health choices if you

If unhappy men were connected to their core selves, they couldn't be abusive, exploitative, or violent toward others—it would go against their core values!

are unplugged from the source—you! Empathy for others and abusing others are incompatible within you.

Your mental health or mental illness directly corelates with your relationship with your core self!

Understanding the full spectrum of your mental health starts with knowing you. Mental health and mental illness focus on the fragmented parts of ourselves or the unified parts of ourselves. This is the fork in the road between becoming healthier or becoming more detached from yourself and your world. Psychological cohesiveness makes sense of all the memories, emotions, thoughts, and fears you have experienced. Fragmentation creates mental and psychological chaos and confusion.

Core Self Questions—The Picture of Me

1. What's my core belief about honesty?
2. What's my core belief about love relationships?
3. What's something in my past that violated my core values?
4. What's my core belief about my health?
5. What's my core belief about my appearance and physical body?

Definition of Your Self-Acceptance

Our self-acceptance is the expression of our core values, opinions of ourselves, our goals, and desires. Compassion for ourselves and for others starts with accepting our "perfectly imperfect" selves. You are courageous to take risks, express your opinions, try new things, start a hobby, begin a morning routine, and share your feelings. These actions feel positive and strengthen you.

Additionally, you have learned to see yourself as separate from others, having boundaries between yourself and others. You embrace differences and recognize that no two people are identical. You are familiar with your dark side and don't reject your moods, emotions, or feelings as "bad." You don't seek other people's validation, approval for how you should think or feel. You have your own ideas about your life and the circumstances surrounding you.

Nothing in your life will ever be accomplished without your involvement. No one can make your life happen or do it for you.

Two points of interest: Perfectionism is a form of self-loathing that leads to self-hatred. Self-acceptance is synonymous with personal growth and change.

Throughout life, you will learn things about yourself that you like or want to change. You have the emotional bandwidth to make improvements to be empathic, compassionate, and accepting. Life experiences can expand our perspectives about ourselves and others—what you do with this information is the question. Impermanence/change is normal, not an issue to control or something to resist. You have your opinions; you do not allow others to tell you what to think or do. You are decisive about taking responsibility for your beliefs, feelings, and choices.

For instance, you enjoy donating clothes that you aren't using to others who might be less fortunate. The action of doing, giving, donating aligns with your core values. Reinforcing your values and desires strengthens your self-image, your internal picture of you. Humility, forgiveness, and generosity are all traits that align with building stronger connections between you and your core values.

> *Anxiety is the result of outsourcing approval.*—Dr. Nicole LePera, psychologist

There are also actions that weaken self-acceptance. Some examples include: lying to your partner and yourself; having a sexual or emotional affair; stealing from your company; withholding information in a business deal; being rude and argumentative; being critical of others; and choosing to be aggressive.

What's interesting about life is that the negative actions or decisions we make impact us. The reality is that we truly are hurting ourselves, even if we don't immediately understand the consequences.

> **You can't outsource your self-accepting process—it's an in-house project, and your sole responsibility to complete.**

We ultimately damage ourselves when we seek revenge, gossip, bully, or embezzle money from our selfish boss. None of these actions strengthens our emotional connections or emotional bonds with ourselves. Your core self is always revealed by the choices you make, which forms the picture you carry emotionally about yourself: *your self-acceptance.*

Anything important in your life requires emotional investment in it and in yourself—no connection, no progress. Psychological connection is the *only* pathway to change and to create your own life.

Self-Acceptance Questions—The Picture of Me

- What's something about myself that I like?
- Who is the person that I show the world versus my private self?

- What is a roadblock in my life that stops me from excelling?
- Who did I imagine I would be as an adult when I was a child?

Definition of Individuation/Separation—Leaving the Mothership

We discussed the various reasons and implications why you can't bring your mother or entire family along in your personal and love life—ultimately it never turns out well. The process of readjusting our primary emotional connections from our childhood and teenage years is inevitable. Sons naturally start to question, wonder, and want to get out of their safe harbor of life.

The task of creating your own personal space is one of the most underrated tasks that men face in their lifetime. Read that again and again. The brotherhood is ruthless when a buddy is a "mama's boy," still under his mother's control and influence. Forming your identity always includes emotional separation from your mothership of comfort.

Frustration tolerance and emotional boundaries are skills developed via creating your own identity.

Emotional aloofness, fear of intimacy, feeling suffocated, sexual dysfunction, and isolating are all symptoms of an incomplete individuation process. Knowing yourself and withstanding the disappointment of important women in your life are invaluable. Learning to be emotionally self-sufficient is a universal masculinity task.

Often, men forgo the discomfort of disappointing their mothers and emotionally "replace" their mothers with a mother proxy. We know that never works—never. It's impossible to thrive in an adult sexual relationship when your partner is either your son or your mother. This is an emotionally incestuous bond that is damaging and ultimately fatal to the relationship. No couple can properly function, communicate, and respect each other with this problematic arrangement for the long term.

Every son has to learn how to function without his mother's emotional support in order to enter into adulthood.

lematic arrangement for the long term.

According to author Robert Bly, in Grimm brothers' mythology, the mother holds the key to the boy's freedom. The boy has to sneak into his mother's chambers and retrieve the key from under her pillow. This key unlocks the gate for his exit from his mother's house. Once he opens the gate, the boy leaves on his masculine journey. The mother holds the key—the permission and control—to the son's masculine courage or failure.

According to the Grimm brothers' mythology stories, the boy never receives his mother's permission to leave, thus he must be courageous and go without her permission, a task many men avoid. The outcome is living in his mother's castle for all the days of his life, unfilled and infantilized.

Pleasing our mothers was encouraged while we were growing up; now as adult men, we have to unlearn that approval seeking and be emotionally self-supporting! This a primary task of becoming a man.

Developing frustration tolerance allows you to have your own opinion, ideas, and choices when your mother or an important woman in your life wants something different. This emotional skill set is highly underrated. Emotional boundaries are the flip side of the coin for frustration tolerance. The ability to know, have, and express your own opinion and choices in the face of contrary opinions is frustration tolerance. Having the conviction to know and pursue what you want is your job to complete.

This isn't selfishness, self-centeredness, or being insensitive; *it's knowing your limits and exercising your boundaries in the face of criticism.* Healthy relationships can tolerate differences without personalizing the issue as an attack. Your personal clarity helps you set and maintain emotional boundaries for yourself and your partner. Codependency, on the other hand, lacks boundaries or awareness of your needs and wants in a relationship.

Codependency is the inability to have a healthy relationship with oneself or others. It's about living through others, rather than living through yourself!

Tolerating the emotional backlash, silent treatment, or upset is a positive side effect of your individuation from the "mothership." The emotional clarity to understand and not to react but rather to respond is empowering. The fear of "caving" to please your mother/family no longer controls you or clouds your judgment. Having a strong, independent relationship with yourself and your partner is preventive medicine for this mother/man-child dynamic.

Domestic violence and all forms of spousal abuse is a desperate attempt to control the other person emotionally, psychologically, and physically.

Domestic violence, spousal abuse, and violent acts against women/partners are fueled by the couple's enmeshment—lack of personal identity. The unspoken belief that neither partner can survive without the other person creates despair and attempts to control your partner. The aggressive reaction to feeling abandoned rapidly escalates into emotional and physical violence to offset the couple's instability. This is why the developmental step of individuating in your masculine journey can't be skipped or dismissed as optional. The research on violent men points to their lack of psychological insight, poor impulse control, enmeshed boundaries, and inability to tolerate disagreements (i.e., no frustration tolerance).

Cautionary Tale—Individuation Gone Wrong

I was referred to an eighteen-year-old high school senior, Luis, who was having difficulty communicating with his mother. Luis was in his last semester of his senior year in high school and was planning to go to college out of state in the fall. These comments are a sample of our therapy sessions.

LUIS: My mother threatens me all the time if I don't agree with her about anything. She constantly accuses me of getting stoned or drunk. When I sober up, she still calls me a liar. Then if I give her some "attitude," she threatens to kill herself because I am ungrateful.

ME: Luis, can you and your mother have a discussion in which you agree to disagree?

LUIS: Hell no, my mother will tell me that she was raped as a teenager, and I should be grateful for all that she does for me and not to question her. What do I say when she screams at me about being raped? I feel so empty inside when we argue because my mom says crazy stuff and I believe she would kill herself if I really yelled at her.

ME: What do you do when the discussion becomes heated and threatening?

LUIS: At some point I just stop talking; I don't say anything, nod my head in agreement, and go to my room. I then play my video games for hours trying to get my anger out.

ME: Sounds like you have the ability to control yourself in these emotionally charged arguments?

LUIS: Well, this is why I am in your office. I finally snapped and told my mother to kill herself and stop threatening me with it. She went to slap me, and I grabbed her hand and told her I would break it off if she slapped me. She backed off. I told her that I wasn't going to be her punching bag anymore. My parents have been divorced for eight years. My mom says when she's angry that I am like my father, a pussy. I told her that I knew why dad left her.

ME: What did your mother do when you challenged her?

LUIS: My mom told me to get the fuck out of the house. I walked to my dad's house, which is five miles away. I have been living with him for the last three weeks. I am never talking to my mother ever again or living with her. I'd rather be homeless than be her slave.

ME: One thing about anger is that it doesn't last forever, and forever is a very long time. Are you talking to your mother at all?

LUIS: I blocked her on my phone, and I let my dad deal with her. I am done and going to college in the fall three thousand miles away from Los Angeles and my mother.

Backstory: Luis gave me permission to meet with his mother and help rebuild communication between the two of them. The mother, Lucy, was angry, resentful, and heartbroken that Luis had rejected her. Lucy is a single mother who left her ex-husband for her college sweetheart eight years ago. Lucy told me that when she was a college freshman, she was raped and has never been the same. Lucy has never gone to any type of mental health treatment or rape support group. I asked Lucy why she threatens to kill herself when she argues with Luis. Lucy feels that threatening to die will make Luis appreciate her.

I explained to Lucy that threatening to commit suicide is a form of emotional blackmail. It doesn't work and breeds only resentment.

Educating the mind without educating the heart is no education at all.—Aristotle

FIVE STEPS TO BUILDING YOU—IT'S YOUR PROJECT

Most people do not really want freedom, because freedom involves responsibility, and most people are frightened of responsibility.
—Sigmund Freud, father of psychology

We discussed the three initial steps in forming your identity, psychological independence, core self, and who you are in your family. We now explore five steps to further form the man you choose to be. Each of these five steps is designed for you to master, apply, and incorporate into your masculine mental health.

- Emotional boundaries—Learning to say "no" before saying "yes"
- Frustration tolerance—Emotional maturity, deactivating your triggers
- Emotional sobriety—Mental clarity, responding not reacting, addictive behaviors

- Acceptance of your (and your family's) DNA—Knowing who and what you are, generational mental health, and family and psychological patterns. What has been psychologically passed on to you?
- Your relationship style—Isolation versus connection: how you connect, relate, and build a secure bond. Who do I become in a romantic union?

EMOTIONAL BOUNDARIES

We discussed this issue several times before and it's worth revisiting during our self-design project. There are many reasons this concept is imperative to your inner development. Your sense of living in the world is knowing the limits that form the parameters of your life. Your psychological, physical, mental, emotional, and personal thoughts and feelings form who and

> *Progress is possible only with change; men who choose not to change their minds, perspectives, or behaviors cannot change anything—including themselves! It's your choice.*

what you are. Boundaries draw a line between two objects, thus forming two individuals. Small children learn about their personal space as a means of understanding how they impact others. Children who have their physical or emotional being violated don't experience the benefit of having their limits respected by adults in their life. Children who grew up in a family with appropriate limit setting know how to respect and maintain their own.

A lump of mashed potatoes doesn't require firm limits. Emotionally, psychologically, and physically contrasting yourself from someone else allows you to experience your own individuality and autonomy. Awareness leads to responsibility for your actions, choices, decisions, goals, and relationships. You have complete responsibility for your life and how it unfolds. No one else controls you or defines you—it's your choice.

> *Until you learn how to say "no," your "yes" is meaningless!*

The first boundary you learned was saying "no." Children have to learn how to say "no" before their "yes" is valid. Your first boundary starts with "no," and it's the boundary that sets all the other limits in your life.

How to Create Boundaries—Four Mandatory Action Steps

Step 1—Learn to say "no" where and when you automatically say "yes." Write down three places, three people, and three situations that are difficult for you to say "no." For the next seven days, practice saying "no" when you don't know what to say. The nine areas you identified are the places to start creating a healthy dividing line between yourself and others. Until you learn how to say "no" in your life, your "yes" will be meaningless! Read that again.

What area or people do you erase yourself and your boundaries for?

Step 2—Pause before answering any request, question, or favor someone asks of you. Pausing allows you to ask yourself what you want to do (or not do). Your boundaries are defined when you know what you want and what you don't want. This applies to picking a restaurant, dessert, clothing to buy, vacation plans, making social plans with your friends, and accepting dinner invitations. Nothing in your life exists without boundaries.

Boundaries are your psychological and physical limits, which are reminders of your value and importance.

Step 3—Decide what is nonnegotiable in your life. What three things in your personal life are nonnegotiable? Second, what three things in your romantic relationship are nonnegotiable? Third, what three things are nonnegotiable in your friendships, your health, with your colleagues, and in your career? Finally, what three things are nonnegotiable in your family? Your core values via your self-acceptance actions are apparent by establishing your boundaries based on your priorities. You have listed twenty-one different areas and situations in which you now have boundaries.

You and your values continue to develop throughout life, therefore establishing new boundaries is part of the adult process.

Step 4—Stop seeking approval by dismissing your priorities, canceling your plans, and not being honest about your circumstances. Give yourself permission to make plans, have your own life, and enjoy friends without getting someone's permission.

FRUSTRATION TOLERANCE

Frustration tolerance is the ability to disengage when your emotional triggers are pushed (or hit with a hammer). Tolerance is the emotional resistance and internal clarity not to personalize or to react during a current disagreement. Self-control and self-restraint to manage your uncomfortable feelings is frustration endurance and emotional stamina, which are aspects of this dynamic.

Having psychological control of how and when you want to respond is a hallmark feature of adult maturity.

Being able to understand and accept another's opinion without arguing is a sign of your emotional and psychological balance.

The following qualities comprise the everyday use of frustration tolerance. It's the emotional component of accepting differences that otherwise can lead to a slippery slope into danger. Rage, anger, and resentment make accepting differences very challenging. Good parenting, mentoring, and being a loving partner is having emotional room to hold, understand, and accept your partners "*disease*." You have the mental capacity to separate yourself from the heated discussion, argument, or debate. Accepting—not avoiding—the uncomfortable feelings allows you to remain objective and emotionally balanced.

Self-love, self-acceptance, and courage are all forms of your core strength, which fosters insight, wisdom, and tolerance for handling difficulties.

These skills were developed within the first year of your life: learning to tolerate a wet diaper and inconsistent feedings, being held by strangers, and being stared at by your siblings. Rather than react emotionally, you sometimes paused and observed what was happening. Your core self is strengthened whenever you exercise your ability to not go "offside." We have to stay on our side, within ourselves, to be helpful, objective, and supportive.

How to Develop Frustration Tolerance

Emotional maturity is another term for frustration tolerance. Shame, trauma, anxiety, fear, and unresolved resentments breed impatience, overreactions, aggressive outbursts, violence, and poor choices.

The "3 Cs" psychological behavioral self-check tool is invaluable for managing guilt. These questions help to manage our feelings of powerlessness and clarify our role and responsibility in any situation or relationship. Using this technique over time strengths your emotional ability to objectively see your role in any situation.

Carrying the "3 Cs" on your mental notecard serves as a reminder of your ability to tolerate and understand your responsibility.

- Did I cause it?
- Can I control it?
- Can I change it?

Asking yourself these three questions when confronting any issue is a productive way to get immediate mental clarity and insight about your role and responsibility. This method helps to reduce anxiety and lower our frustration about things we know we can't control.

Understanding your boundaries, responsibilities, and actions that must be taken breeds humility and calmness. The natural by-product of emotionally knowing what you need to do eliminates the guesswork from any situation. You can manage your feelings, emotions, and reactions with firsthand knowledge of what is needed.

> *If you wouldn't say it to a friend, don't say it to yourself.*
> —Jane Travis, therapist

EMOTIONAL SOBRIETY

Is your psychological balance sober and consistent or unpredictable and reactive? When you are physically intoxicated, stoned, angry, avoidant, or on some type of pain pill cloud, your mental and emotional reactions and functions are impaired. You can get physically sober from most drugs within four to six weeks. The hard part is rewiring your brain not to react, crave, and avoid taking responsibility. The ingrained psychological patterns of being enraged, avoidant, reckless, and pleasure seeking are hinderances to any degree of mental health or quality of life.

Emotional Intoxication and Why It Matters

Any type of exaggerated response is a sign that our shame and past traumas are slipping into our present day. When we separate/individuate, connect with our core self, and engage our self-accepting beliefs, we can stay calm and even minded.

Mental clarity is only possible when the emotional waters of your mind are calm and balanced—emotional sobriety breeds clarity!

Crazy thoughts, immature reactions, and childish beliefs, petty reactions, revengeful ideas, and losing control of yourself because of your anger are all forms of emotional intoxication. The psychology of addiction recovery's fundamental premise is that three things will change your behavior: legal intervention (i.e., arrest), you, or death! The first two wakeup calls lead to change. The third alternative is harsh and sadly very accurate.

Remaining Emotionally Sober

Exposing the myths of your emotional distortions and creating a positive rebuttal with a positive narrative helps you to remain emotionally sober. Please write down your answers and thoughts to all of the following questions.

1. What in your life feels unfair, wrong, or upsetting?
2. What settings, people, and moods cause you to feel uneasy and to emotionally check out?
3. Rebut your negative self-talk. For instance, if you hate being judged by others, your rebuttals might be: "I choose to understand myself and take full responsibility for the things I do." "Choosing to be gracious to myself and not to reject my own feelings feels really good." "No one judges me as hard as I judge myself."

ACCEPTANCE OF YOUR AND YOUR FAMILY'S DNA

Your family of origin is your starting line on your journey; it is not your finish line or destiny in life. You decide your destiny and who you choose to be. The DNA you inherited is more than your physical appearance, strengths, and eye color. The most important thing to embrace is your family's psychological legacy via the emotional DNA transmission process.

> *Your DNA is more than your looks and physicality; it's also a combination of the emotional and psychological legacy issues passed on to you!*

According to the founding fathers of family therapy from the late 1940s and 1950s, emotional illness can be passed down through the family's emotional style of relating. If trauma, personality problems, and masculinity issues aren't addressed in the current generation, the dysfunction is passed along. Over time, the issues, personality problems, and mental health challenges increase in severity with each subsequent generation. This process is known as the family transgenerational transmission process.

> *Your family's mental health issues are a starting point, not your emotional ending point.*

Positive qualities, characteristics, strengths can also be passed along via this natural psychological family tree.

Throughout the generations of a family, unresolved trauma, physical abuse (via war or sexual molestation), and family secrets of shame and denial become increasingly more problematic. The horrors that families bury but can't erase from their psychological legacy are as serious as your great-grandfather's untreated cancer.

Know your emotional family history of trauma, sexual abuse, addiction, incarceration, mental illness, wealth and prosperity, and the positive qualities that have been passed along to you. These factors are part of the fabric of your mental health history and life today. Men typically are embarrassed about their parents, siblings, financial status, neighborhood, or physical appearance. The biggest DNA secret in your family is the psychological issues that have been handed down without question, treatment, or concern. What do you know about both sides of your parents' mental health legacies?

The term generational wealth is not limited to financial inheritance; it includes your mental health strengths and challenges handed down from prior generations. Until recently, mental health, psychology, therapy, and self-help support groups were few and far between.

Your mental health care is a proactive change in your life and in the generations that follow you. Your entire life is a composite of many factors. The following list of questions is a starting point for you to talk to your parents, aunts, uncles, cousins, and anyone else who knows the private story of your family. This information, I guarantee, will be enlightening and helpful in understanding more about your struggles and genetic predispositions.

Your Family's Mental Health Inventory

- Does depression, anxiety, avoidance, denial, and shame run in our family?
- What is a family secret that is known but never spoken about?
- Does your family address the issues of violence or any type of abuse?
- What's your primary mental health challenge?
- What is a masculinity issue or strength you share with the men in your family?

YOUR RELATIONSHIP STYLE—ATTACHMENT, VULNERABILITY, AND COMMITMENT

We discussed how intimate relationships are the most unique and special relationships you have in your life. Being a parent, brother, son, colleague, cousin, and friend are all very important connections. No other relationship in your life is on the same level as your romantic relationship. This is the only relationship in which you can explore your childhood; ask for your needs and desires to be met; heal; and be supportive, transparent, and completely vulnerable emotionally and psychologically.

Your Preexisting Relationship Influences—Carrying Your Own Baggage

Who we choose and why. Our unresolved parental conflict, wounds, or needs are strong, unconscious magnets that draw us to our partners. Which of your parents are you angry at or resentful about?

Our love language is our unmet emotional needs from our childhood! Read this sentence again. Each time we accuse our partners of being insensitive or unloving, it's important to consider our own preexisting emotional attachment in the matter. Our experience of feeling loved, cared for, and understood guides how we interact romantically. Knowing your attachment style and desires allows you to learn about theirs.

Our partners mirror the issues we need to address in our own lives. Many times, our partners' shortcomings are similar to our own, and that is why we become irritated with them. Our partners are living reminders of what we need to heal.

Five Marriage Factors

The factors below, along with our preexisting personal issues, are instrumental in selecting a partner. The more insight you have into your emotional self, the greater opportunity to find the type of partner you can build a life with. There isn't a masculine quality or trait that will not be important in your long-term relationship. How you express yourself starts with the type of relationship you cocreate.

- *Feeling special*—You and your partner are emotionally connected, vulnerable, and honest with one another. Feeling seen, heard, and appreciated creates a sense of specialness that each of you feels. Knowing that you matter to your partner removes any jealousy or pettiness about past relationships.
- *Feeling understood*—Your personality, unique talents, jokes, sense of humor, and serious side are acceptable and welcomed by your partner. You extend the same courtesy to your partner so the two of you can thrive in an atmosphere of acceptance. You discuss disagreements without personalizing the issue. Feeling understood takes time and patience as your partner learns your "backstory" of who you are today.
- *Feeling loved and forgiven*—There is emotional safety and tenderness that allows you to be perfectly imperfect. There is the absence of criticism or verbal berating for making mistakes. Your relationship is your safe place

in life. You show respect by listening to your partner's concerns, honoring his or her need for space, and expressing his or her opinions. These types of gestures put "emotional money" into the couple's psychological bank account.

- *Intimate communication*—Your sexual and physical attraction is mutual and complementary. The kindness expressed outside the bedroom translates directly into the bedroom. Maintaining a sexual relationship improves the quality of all the other forms of communication between you and your partner. Kindness breeds sexual desire. Anger breeds isolation and loss of emotional connection and safety. The way in which you speak to your partner indicates how they feel about you. Kindness breeds intimacy. Harshness breeds isolation.
- *Transparency/vulnerability:* These are two different issues yet similar. Transparency is not withholding or keeping pertinent information secret about your life, such as having children with another partner whom you never married. Vulnerability is having insight into yourself and your partner. You have the psychological capacity to express empathy to your partner. He or she feels heard, understood, and cared for by your attention.

SUMMARY—WHAT IS THE PICTURE YOU CARRY IN YOUR WALLET OF YOURSELF?

The six traits for developing your love life and carrying your own baggage include your four horsemen in your adult world of relationships. We are designed genetically to attach, bond, love, and experience living our lives as we choose. This entire chapter is dedicated to your discovery and use of all your tools, insights, and wisdom to continue to build and create the life you choose. You are building the man within you; no one else is; it's all you.

The three steps of awakening your core self (core awareness, self-acceptance, individuation/separation) and the five steps of your identity (emotional boundaries, tolerance, sobriety, accepting and knowing your family's DNA, and your relationship process) are the lumber with which you construct your life with going forward. You have the blueprints with your life plans and goals in your hands.

One question that I ask my clients is: "What emotional picture do you have of yourself deep inside your heart?" That picture of your younger self is important to never lose or to disconnect from. The pictures we hold of ourselves in childhood and adolescence reveal what we feel and believe about ourselves deep down.

What does the picture you carry from childhood look like? How old is he? What's he wearing? Kids are adorable and so were you as a child. Finally, what would you like to say to the younger you about your life?

> *Being both soft and strong is a combination very few have mastered.*—Unknown

CHAPTER SIXTEEN

CHANGE, FORGIVENESS, AND YOUR FIVE F-BOMBS

Being Your Own Man

Out of suffering have emerged the strongest souls. The most massive characters are seared with scars.—Khalil Gibran

Our brains are wired for connections; trauma rewires them for protection. That's why healthy relationships are difficult for wounded people.—Ryan North, therapist

The curious paradox is that when I accept myself just as I am then I can change.—Carl Rogers, founding father of psychology

The weak can never forgive. Forgiveness is the attribute of the strong.—Gandhi

MEN'S MENTAL HEALTH AND PERSONALITY ISSUES— REMOVING YOUR ROADBLOCKS

We discussed throughout the book the challenges of developing the four main aspects of our masculinity (physical, emotional, relational, and personal) and the understanding necessary to accomplish your building of the man within you. Now we discuss some common roadblocks, personality issues, and barriers that you have created. It takes courage to change, to forgive and understand yourself. The alternative—avoidance—leads to despair. Men want to embrace masculinity in a new way that empowers them to be better men, partners, friends, colleagues, husbands, fathers, sons, and a good neighbor to the new people down the street. *Men want to feel better about being men!*

In order to get where we want to go, we must remove our self-imposed psychological roadblocks, old-school "dude" thinking and "jerk" behavior, which stops productive lasting change. Many of the poor behaviors that men engage in aren't just momentary lapses in judgment but personality problems. The psychological bottom line: your personality either draws people to you or keeps them away.

Men who amend their personality blind spots tap into their potential.

Think about that for a minute. Does your personality "energy" attract people to you and make them interested in you and want to spend time with you? Or is your personality rough around the edges, irritable at times, or moody? You already know the answers to these questions. The next question is: are you willing to be emotionally insightful and address your father-son issues, respond to your partner with compassion, and widen your perspective on yourself in order to experience peace of mind? Of course, the answer is yes, but how do you make changes to these ingrained behaviors and your personality? Let's start by looking at your personality blind spots and what can be amended.

What Is a Personality Disorder?

Do I have a personality disorder? Let's first define personality disorder before discussing whether you have "touches" of one or a full-blown diagnosis. The following definition is from the *Diagnostic and Statistical Manual of Mental Disorders*, which states:

> A personality disorder is an enduring pattern of inner experience and behavior that deviates markedly from the expectations of the individual's culture, is pervasive and inflexible, has an onset in adolescents or early adulthood, is stable over time and leads to distress or impairment. (American Psychiatric Association 2015, 645)

The development of our personalities becomes more consistent, predictable, and expressive of ourselves with age. By the time we reach our late teens and early twenties, we have established regular patterns of interacting with our friends socially and interpersonally. It's important to note that any personality type can be amended and healed to be less problematic in your life.

We aren't discussing organic disorders that are genetic and relate to brain abnormalities outside of a person's control. This would include severe head trauma from concussions that adversely affect a person's functioning and perception of their world (e.g., severe delusionary thought disorders, auditory and visual hallucinations). These are not the roadblocks that 95 percent of men struggle with or face. These disorders require psychiatric care and medication to monitor the symptoms.

This is why the internal picture you carry of yourself is a relevant factor in how you move about in your life. The clarity, awareness, and understanding of yourself enables you to live your life with meaning and purpose. The alternative is a lack of understanding, avoiding your desires, ignoring your intuition, and disconnecting from what you want in life. The lack of self-awareness leads to personality disorders, relationship issues, and professional challenges ranging from mild to severe. The good news is that you can amend and courageously address your personality needs and wounds and feel complete rather than emotionally deprived.

COMMON MALE PERSONALITY TRAITS— ROADBLOCKS WITHIN YOU!

Based on my experience of working with men during the last forty years in professional and clinical settings, I need to address some truisms about the brotherhood. Many of the points below challenge the old-school, psychologically dismissive masculinity. The "old boys club" is giving way to the new school of masculinity, which embodies insight and emotional balance.

- Men can be "jerks" and sensitive simultaneously.
- Men tend to avoid emotional situations and prefer to "fix" them.
- Men can be sexual and depressed at the same time.
- Men carry the heavy burden of trying to be "financial superstars" for their families.
- Men judge other men based on their ability to make money.
- Women want men who have a balanced masculine and feminine emotional awareness.
- Men have feelings and emotions that seem perplexing and confusing to them but not to their partner.
- More and more men are seeking therapy as a means of translating their feelings and understanding their lives.
- Men do better in relationships—all areas of their life benefit.
- Men need strong partners who have boundaries and who will not tolerate their "bad boy" behavior.
- Men avoid discussing their sexual abuse, molestations, and childhood traumas until they can't hide from them any longer.

- Men need their male buddies to recharge their "guy energy" and focus.
- Playing and watching sports are emotional outlets for men and ways to connect with other men.
- Relationships matter to men.
- Having a daughter freaks men out.
- Men personalize divorce as being "defective."
- Men scare men with their anger, aggression, and shame-driven violence.

These statements about men are general and specific. Men have personality issues that block them from excelling and becoming the men they want to be. The following five personality barriers are all treatable and related to the statements above.

While reading the descriptions of the personality barriers below, circle the qualities that describe your behaviors at home, work, socially and with your buddies. There are no wrong answers. Unless we are willing to be honest and acknowledge our self-defeating actions, attitudes, and beliefs, no amount of awareness of our core selves will overcome these brick walls in our lives. Recognizing the traits in yourself is a huge step toward amending and changing them. You may have traits in all five personality sections; however, one category will be the most prominent in your perceptions and reactions to how you live.

Without awareness there is no change.

*Borderline-Angry Personality Behaviors—*Common traits include: insecurity about self; superficial attachments and friendships; fearful of rejection, real or imagined; unable to maintain stable relationships with self or others; irrational mood swings; blames others for personal issues; emotionally connects only through sex; believes everyone hates them or wants to hurt them; lack of trust for self or others; creates "drama" as a means of feeling important; seeks revenge when offended or slighted; prone to violence when scared or emotionally out of control/dysregulated; seeks emotional highs rather than emotional stability; denies unresolved trauma; demanding and impatient; believes in his superiority over others; unable to manage finances or any type of adult responsibilities; seeks a "free ride" in life; dishonest with self and others; avoids accountability; physical appearance is supremely important; high-conflict relationship style; vindictive and prone to revenge to offset feeling powerless; lacks a life purpose and plan.

*Narcissistic Personality, Self-Centered Tendencies—*Common traits include: a deep unconscious sense of inadequacy, which he conceals by devaluing others; believes he is special and that the rules don't apply to him; entitled and seeks special privileges; verbally abusive to others to feel better about himself; unable to be generous unless it serves him; no regard for others' feelings or needs; publicly kind and privately abusive and dangerous; seeks control to feel empowered at the expensive of others; status driven; appearance is everything; unethical behaviors; self-serving decisions; unable to see his role in a conflict; lacks insight and psychological tools and resists vulnerability and transparency; refuses to accept responsibility for his role in a conflict or misunderstanding; lacks compassion and empathy for others; uses others for personal gain and status; directs all conversation back to himself; emotionally and financially withholding; rude and insensitive to subordinates; views people as objects; abusive childhood with unresolved abuse; immature behaviors; no genuine friendships; privately very lonely and sad; viewed as a narcissist by his partner; doesn't allow anyone to see his vulnerability including his partner.

Anxiety Issues, Avoidant Personality—Common traits include: chronic fear of the unknown; seeks reassurance for decisions, choices, and future events; uses self-medicating drugs; unresolved childhood trauma; fears unpredictable situations; chaotic family background; believes that the world is unsafe; tries to control everything and everyone in his world; struggles with boundary issues; controlling behaviors consume his energy; has enmeshed relationships; lacks generosity and feels deprived; obsesses over impending doom scenarios; unable to be emotionally or mentally present; seeks emotional security whenever he is outside of his comfort zone; has a small circle of friends; averse to any type of new experience or situation; resists change; avoids people or new situations; inflexible, adheres to routine; expects people to come to him; life is driven by the unconscious need to be safe; emotional deprivation issues; never feels complete; procrastinates; unable to make decisions small or large; indecisive; lacks generosity; unable to focus on inner personal issues; lives in the past or the future; not comfortable with self or others; depends on others to initiate socializing; refuses to take trips to new destinations; greedy; verbally insensitive; lacks the ability to be intimate with his partner on any level.

A Cautionary Tale—Anxiety Combined with Codependency

ROCCO: I am unsure if I want to marry Heather. We have been dating for two years and she will be thirty-four years old later this year, and she wants children. I also would like to have children; that isn't a problem or concern. I can't imagine my life without her, but she is so anxious and pushy with me. Heather tells me how to drive, literally how to walk, and has to be in control. It drives me crazy.

ME: What keeps you from letting Heather know your thoughts and feelings?

ROCCO: I don't want to upset her. She gets very hurt when I point out things that bother me or that she does that are controlling. Heather thinks that I don't love her because I am not always happy with her.

ME: Avoiding conflict is a short-term solution to a long-term crisis you are creating. Expressing your concerns in a calm manner with respect is what couples do to become connected. Heather has no idea that you are thinking of breaking up with her because of her anxiety issues. You owe her the courtesy of being honest so she can be aware of your concerns and reservations. The only way any of us changes is by knowing how we are impacting the people around us whom we love.

ROCCO: I think Heather knows something is off because we have stopped having sex. Growing up, my mother was a monster. She would either scream at me or be nice. I never knew what I was going to get or be in trouble for. I waited for her reaction before I would speak or do anything. She was scary. I still avoid her [Rocco is thirty-three years old]. I guess I am doing this with Heather. I just don't want her to get mad or upset with me. I know this sounds ridiculous, but it's how I think.

Backstory: Rocco is an only child. His parents divorced when he was ten years old. Rocco's mother didn't want him to see his father after the divorce. Rocco's parents, both before and after the divorce, engaged in heated verbal fights that often resulted in throwing knives and bottles at each other.

Rocco learned at an early age how to placate both his parents. Now as an adult, Rocco is terrified of conflict in a romantic relationship. Rocco's childhood fear of feeling emotionally engulfed or mentally paralyzed is his primary relationship model and a barrier to being vulnerable. Rocco is a retired major league baseball player. He had the reputation among his teammates and coaches as the peacekeeper. Rocco has known Heather since college. They have dated on and off during the last twelve years. Rocco works as a college baseball scout for his former MLB team and is gone six months out of the year. Rocco loves his job and not being tied down to an office.

ROCCO, TWO WEEKS LATER: I broke up with Heather last week. I need to see if I am marrying her because she wants me to or because I really want to. I can't tell the difference, and that's why I took a break. Heather is heartbroken but she knows I struggle with vulnerability issues.

Bipolar (Depression) Disorder—Common traits include: a cynical attitude about his life and the future; views events as either super-positive or dark and hopeless; wakes up depressed or happy—no rhythm to moods; negative outlook about people; socially isolated; prone to heavy drinking or drug use; self-pity about how his life has turned out; verbally hostile toward partner or close friends; blames others for perceived misfortunes; thinks about suicide when feeling powerless; refuses mental health treatment; feels victimized in his career; low physical and emotional energy; poor hygiene; unable to maintain appropriate health habits; poor eating habits; not physically active; low sex drive or hypersexual; can be engaging when energized; uncommunicative with people; avoids any type of medical treatments; acts out anger with cutting his body or excessive tattoos; history of poor mental health; refuses medication; self-medicates with smoking nicotine or marijuana; struggles with feelings of despair and hopelessness; poor work history; difficult personality to have a relationship; blames his problems, choices on his parents; dependent on family or others for financial support; believes there is no cure for his condition; can be charming and friendly then moody and irritable.

Personality Changes Due to Medical Conditions, Grief, Personal Crisis— Common traits include: struggles with aging; irritable and unhappy; laid off at work; no job prospects; can't pay rent or mortgage; being sued; loss of support group; wife left him; struggling with a severe personal medical crisis; cancer survivor; physical mobility is limited; grieving the death of a friend; struggling with child's health crisis; partner had a miscarriage; parents died; financial pressures; overwhelmed by career and family demands; sexual dysfunctions; weight gain; poor self-image; feeling lost in his career; unable to maintain romantic relationship; death of pet; estranged from family, children, or partner; overcoming drug addiction; feeling defective or not good enough; physically aggressive; untreated adult attention deficit issues; in couples therapy; retirement planning issues; late onset of diabetes; empty nest; feels "left behind" by partner; overwhelmed with the therapy process.

NOW WHAT? TREATMENT FOR OUR ROADBLOCKS

Each of these five roadblocks can be removed or at least minimized in your life by applying the five self-accepting steps discussed in the last chapter: connecting with our core self; setting emotional boundaries, maintaining emotional sobriety, developing emotional tolerance, and accepting your family's DNA and your relationship style. Each personality issue can benefit from exposing the wound, accepting it, and changing your response to these old issues when they arise in the present day.

Personality patterns, ingrained habits, and negative thinking can change because they are all fluid interactions. No personality characteristic is permanent unless we choose to allow it to do so. In the past, psychologists have argued that certain personalities are fixed and can't be changed or amended. Today that clinical view is now being questioned because research on neuroplasticity shows how our brain connections can change. The brain can create new neurological pathways, new ways of responding, and increase psychological awareness. Your actual brain and nerve pathways are flexible to change.

> *Bones can heal themselves; skin constantly replaces itself; the brain can make new connections thanks to the neuroplasticity; lungs can generate healthy cells when someone quits smoking.*
> —Allison Futterman

This medical observation by Dr. Futterman shows the incredible resiliency of our mind and body to adapt and regenerate. When men say that they can't change or that "you can't teach an old dog new tricks," this is code for "I don't want to change." These are two different perspectives with two different outcomes. My professional experience has been that resisting change is not about the possibility of not changing but rather about the fear of changing. You wouldn't have read this book thus far if you didn't want to change or at least consider the option. (The other gentlemen who aren't changing as of today gave their copies of this book to their partners to read.)

Your life has been a series of experiences, hopefully more positive than upsetting. Everything we do—from getting up in the morning, going somewhere, walking the dog, having lunch with our partners, the list is endless—comprise the experiences of our lives. All these activities, in our minute-to-minute life journey, display our personality.

Psychologists believe that all your life events, big or small, are viewed, understood, and experienced through your internal values, beliefs, and emotional filters. A poignant analogy about how anxiety, childhood trauma, unresolved resentments, and mental health issues can distort and impair our ability to reach our potential clarifies this point: Emotions follow your thoughts like baby ducks follow their mothers. That doesn't mean the mother knows where she is going!

The five personality types we have discussed all react to this cognitive behavioral response cycle. Dr. Albert Ellis created and developed the universal experience cycle, a four-step sequence for responding to our life events. This process of experiencing the world and forming our thoughts, feelings, and ideas about our life started before we could remember. This brain sequence of living is universal. The cycle of living, of experiencing things, is always interpreting what you do, where you go, what you feel, and how you think: event ➜ thought ➜ feeling ➜ behavior.

Your childhood, as you know, played a critical role in shaping and forming your internal psychological framework, your view of your world, yourself, and the important people in your life. Don't panic if your early years were chaotic, unpredictable, abusive, or if you can't remember them. Your core-self processing center remembers your old beliefs, negative thoughts, and childhood fears and responds to events in your life today. Think about that for a second. Spilling your coffee this morning, running late for an appointment, or being reprimanded for a mistake with a client are seen and experienced through your cognitive software from twenty years ago.

Another analogy is wondering why your first handheld cell phone from 1985 doesn't operate well or connect to the internet today. The reason your phone can't meet the demands of your life today is that when it was manufactured, the internet hadn't been invented yet.

Gentlemen, do not make the mistake of thinking that you have arrived at the pinnacle of your life; it's a process and change is your superpower. What worked for you in high school

Our thinking in our adult life needs to be updated.

doesn't necessarily work well for you today. No one expects a cell phone from the 1980s to operate or function with the capabilities of a present-day smartphone. The same holds true of our cognitive and psychological response cycles, emotional interpretations, or psychological insights. It's time to update our "selves." But not with liposuction or cosmetic surgery: these are internal updates for your masculine maturity.

Think about your response cycle to something that you recognize as an old pattern of anger, frustration, or an unproductive reaction. Write down the event and the thoughts, feelings, and behaviors that event triggers for you. It's not your best or most mature self. Knowing how you feel about certain things isn't wrong or incorrect. The problem is when no other option, opportunity, or perspective is considered. Living inside a psychological vacuum eventually leads to emotional stagnation and mental suffocation. The rigidity of your fixed response cycle, which becomes your belief system, is how your emotional roadblocks, personality issues, and disorders develop. This closed system in your thinking isn't healthy. Rigid thinking and fixed opinions are dangerous to our emotional health and overall quality of life.

Should you choose to be kind or to be right? Choose kindness, and you will always be right!

The quotes above and below illustrate a paradox: what is soft is strong! Personality disorders, relationship issues, and romantic problems are caused by emotional inflexibility, static input, fixed opinions, and outdated perspectives. Our psychological rigidity circumvents our personal growth, personality changes, and maturity. Rigidity, stubbornness, self-righteousness, and fearfulness create mental health and psychological problems. It's impossible to stop the flow of your life without adverse side effects.

Our roadblocks and defensiveness can be likened to being locked in a sixteen-year-old's psychological perspective for life—an endless cycle of frustration and suffering.

No one wants to be a sixteen-year-old forever— this is why change is valuable.

Developing your emotional flexibility as an adult man will serve you well all the days of your life. Flexibility isn't the lack of boundaries and values, rather it's the ability to see other peoples' perspectives, to consider new information, and to be open-minded about being wrong! Men who are always right always will be wrong for refusing to consider the alternative. All the personality types discussed so far share this trait of nongrowth.

> *Water is fluid, and soft and yielding. But water will wear away rock, which is rigid and cannot yield. As a rule, whatever is fluid, soft, and yielding will overcome whatever is rigid and hard. This is another paradox: What is soft is strong.*—Lao Tzu

In order to move past our childhood wounds, adolescent beliefs, and immature reactions, we have to walk back into our history. This journey is not for the purpose of blaming, finger-pointing, or shifting our responsibilities; it's to understand our blind spots and our resistance to certain things and to learn how to move forward. Feeling empty, unnoticed, anxious, "not good enough," unlovable, and not unsafe in the world have a residual impact on us today.

There are four areas that will help you to better understand your experience of how you perceive events, situations, and unpredictable occurrences, which were formed early in your life. Understanding your four psychological response dynamics helps you to be less rigid and fearful, more emotionally flexible, and amenable to new things in your life.

Four Problems in Our Thinking

Minimizing situations, discounting your feelings, ignoring your mental and physical health and significant life changing experiences—For instance, in chapter 10, a young boy comes home from school and is told that his dog died. His mother says "sorry" and walks out of the room. That little boy learned to minimize his loss and to ignore his feelings and the importance of his relationship to his core self. Sammy, in chapter 7, whose father and neighbor were both killed in front of him on a Saturday afternoon, never considered the magnitude of this terrifying experience. Sammy's fiancée refused to marry him unless he came to therapy. Sammy finally acknowledged the severity of the trauma caused by his father's death.

The emotional disconnection minimizes important events and experiences for you. The result is that you learn that your emotions, feelings, and psychological insights are trivial and not important. Instead, you became aloof, withdrawn, and without insight into yourself and others. Eventually, your unmet needs create an emotional wall around you. Many years later, the wall becomes a personality issue, disorder, or a major hindrance to your quality of life.

Selective abstraction/distortions—This is our inability to accurately perceive ourselves without shaming, criticizing, and overemphasizing our weaknesses. This is the damaged inner mirror through which you view life. It distorts your career, relationships, and your body image. The emotional distortion can become very serious and lead to developing a paranoid personality. Your mental distortion believes that everyone and everything means to harm you. This isn't true but it feels that way. You live as if your world is constantly under attack.

As a child, you can convince yourself that there is a huge monster in your bedroom closet at night. Your parents open the closet door and turn on the light, revealing the scary monster to be the shadow of a yellow raincoat on a hanger. You see this raincoat and realize that you can distort and misinterpret people, things, and situations. Our fears and traumas skew our emotional feedback loop of proper processing and understanding events and scary situations.

Learning to "reality test" your assumptions keeps you from magnifying a flaw or self-doubt into a major problem or life-threatening belief or event. Focus on your strengths and what you can do rather than on what you can't do. The mental shift from being fearful to taking action is the antidote to your distorted relationships, career, and family. Men need the brotherhood to bounce ideas off and to get constructive feedback and support for our concerns and fears.

Magnification—This is about making "mountains out of molehills." Selective thinking and processing is focused on potential threats and problems to your security and safety, and it's situationally driven. There is underlying anxiety or hysteria within you that believes any problem can be the "end." The question remains, the end of what?

Unresolved childhood beliefs are carried just below the surface of your life. For example, you fear that a misstep with your boss could result in termination; you have a headache, which could be a brain tumor; your child is upset about a school friend, and you call the parents to resolve their issue. You grew up in a house where things were unpredictable and something bad was going to happen. The lack of physical and emotional security created your fight-or-flight response to minor events and the magnification of nonevents. Your perspective and view of life are influenced and controlled by your unresolved fears and heartbreaks as a young boy. If you distract yourself with a crisis, then you don't have to look at yourself or be uncomfortable.

You seem be controlled and unemotional about situations at work or with your family, but underneath you vibrate with anxiety, fear, and uncertainty. Magnifying trivial issues is a psychological self-protective mechanism for avoiding—not dealing with or addressing—the deeper traumas in your life. Chronic worry about impending doom and negative imaginary scenarios keeps you from feeling or thinking about what is happening in your marriage, with your kids, or your poor health. This unconscious emotional tool is a powerful protection device that is resistant to change. The physical rush of adrenaline, the excited brain chemistry, and the feelings of empowerment create patterns that disrupt our mental health balance.

Magnifying events and experiences and misinterpreting situations prevent you from calming yourself and remaining objective and nonreactive, which isolates you from your personal issues.

Catastrophizing—This takes magnifying to a higher level of panicking, attention seeking, crisis management, and need to be needed. Rarely in life are there true, full-blown catastrophes. Ninety-nine percent of the time, you are overreacting to life events with underlying emotional need of being "seen" and accepted.

Men who adopt this coping skill in childhood experience an endless cycle of gloom and doom scenarios. You developed feelings of despair as a response to your chaotic and unpredictable childhood. As children, we experience life without a filter or any preexisting knowledge or tools to manage the adults in our life. The emotional "drama" you witnessed became the foundation on which you experience and understand your life. The exaggeration of a personal event, relationship issue, or something that happened this morning is flavored with your underlying panic of living, being a man, a partner, a parent, and any position of responsibility. Life secretly scares you and you would like to hide but you can't.

Any event—from a parking ticket to a prostate cancer diagnosis—all register at the same level of emotional and mental severity. Your psychological filter for understanding events is skewed in the direction of disaster. The mental health perspectives of calmness and peace of mind aren't on your radar screen. There is always something pending that is going to ruin or harm your life. Your catastrophic belief in life is your biggest challenge! The mental exhaustion with which you are constantly living due to your heightened state of alert and cognitive panic is connected to your family of origin.

These four cognitive distortions are part of the reason men have been resistant to emotional vulnerable, empathy, and the sensitive feminine side of their masculinity. The four qualities of your core self can begin to help you shift your mantra of life from fear—my world is on fire—to calmness, patience, security, and the belief that things work out.

Your emotional insight can offset these four psychological barriers to your personal growth. Incorporating new elements of emotional safety into your old behavioral patterns, reactions, and beliefs yields a newer perspective of you. Overcoming the lack of emotional insight and awareness will stop the cycle of minimizing yourself and your life. Emotional clarity, mental acuity, and psychological stability are by-products of responding to life without old resentments clouding your judgment.

Emotional sobriety is your self-regulation to triggering events from the past, people who irritate you, and your own issues. Clarity and sobriety reduce the distortion of selective abstraction in your thinking, choices, and behavior. Letting go of your past allows you to stay in the present moment. You can't be in two places at once! You tried but it didn't work. What happens is that you become fragmented and split between two worlds.

FORGIVENESS—WE ALL NEED IT

Holding a grudge doesn't make you strong. It makes you bitter. Forgiveness doesn't make you weak. It sets you free.—Unknown

The process of forgiveness is a commonly misunderstood term and concept. The greatest act of kindness, self-love, and concern for your life is detaching it from your wounds, resentments, revengeful thoughts, and hatred. The quote above is a universal truth that transcends all cultural, ethnic, economic, and educational groups, and it is your personal story.

Your past isn't all bad or negative; rather, it's a mixture of many different emotional variables: trauma, tragic events, awkward situations, themes of neglect, family emotional style, and you. It's these particular points or events that you can choose to release and move your life past them.

Men are often defined by the abusive father they had growing up. Unless those emotional and psychological wounds are resolved, that boy is now a walking wounded adult man with a lifetime of resentment inside of him. Worse case, this man is the "walking dead" emotionally, relationally, and personally. His eyes are open, but the soul in this man is dying. All the parts of your life are impacted by the resentments you hold or let go. The mind-body connection, as we discussed earlier, is the case in point here. Your body can't ignore or pretend that your emotions, feelings, and beliefs are holding resentment and disdain. Everything in your life is connected and related.

> *Change requires our detaching from the past, no longer living there!*

The first step for any type of trauma recovery requires letting go, detaching from the person or event, and forgiving yourself. The second is detaching from the circumstances and giving the person another chance to be in your life. These two types of healing are as critical to your mental health as oxygen is critical to your life.

A Cautionary Tale—Abuse, Mental Illness, and Acceptance

The following vignette is about a family mental health issue that wasn't understood or properly treated until many years later. Eric is thirty-four years old and his brother, Gary, is two years younger. Eric came to see me because he and his wife are having a baby, and Eric is adamant that he doesn't want his brother around the baby.

ERIC: My brother growing up was a monster. He was unmedicated bipolar with an explosive-impulsive personality. When I would babysit him, Gary would get mad at me, kick down my bedroom door, and try to strangle me. My mother is also bipolar and refused medication until I was fifteen years old. My father threatened to divorce her if she didn't get medical treatment. Once my mom was on medication, my relationship with her dramatically improved. She was calm, reasonable, and emotionally stable. My brother, now at age thirty-two, still messes around with his medication.

ME: Eric, how is your relationship with your brother now that you both are adults not living together? [Gary lives in Wisconsin for work.]

ERIC: Terrible. Gary is still a steamroller whenever we talk. I am off the phone within ten minutes of speaking with him. I haven't seen Gary since my father's funeral seven years ago. My wife and I deliberately eloped five years ago so I wouldn't have to deal with my family or brother.

ME: Are you scared of your brother?

ERIC: Yes, I am still seeing him as a crazy teenager trying to strangle me or light the house on fire. My brother could have killed all of us a dozen times if he wasn't stopped. Gary is better when he is on his medication. He is calmer, approachable, and not aggressive or hostile toward me. He asks me all the time to come see him and hang out.

ME: Eric, having untreated mental illness is debilitating and destructive to the individual and to their family. You know that your brother had no control over his chemical imbalance, bizarre behaviors, and impulsive urges. Gary didn't choose to be a terrorist. This was a medical issue that required psychiatric treatment. Could you think about your brother as someone who is suffering rather than a monster?

ERIC: I have never looked at my brother from the perspective that he wasn't willfully trying to harm me. The idea that his illness wasn't his choice or fault is interesting. When he finally got on medication in high school, Gary did much better in school and socially. Now he is married and has two young boys whom I have never met.

ME: Eric, have you ever considered forgiving your brother for your and his childhood trauma and craziness?

ERIC: Never have thought of that either. My brother is always Gary, and someone I passionately avoid.

Eric has come to a major fork in the road: he must choose whether to forgive and have no relationship with Gary or forgive and let Gary back into his life.

First Type of Forgiveness—You

You're disconnecting from that event, circumstance, or person. Creating emotional distance allows you to close that chapter in your book. It doesn't mean forgetting about it or pretending it didn't happen. The disconnection unplugs its influence, and it no longer controls your life. Let the connection go and acknowledge the situation so that it's not a factor in your relationships. Our goal is for you to put the past on the shelf and start writing a new chapter in your life. All sorts of mental health issues begin with our constant recycling, replaying, and rereading our trauma. Oftentimes our identity is associated with our victimization.

The field of psychology uses many different words for the word "forgiveness." The various words all lead back to the same place: you and your resentment. The point is that to the degree that you accept and forgive yourself and the people in your past or present day is the same degree to which you will heal, love, and have a fulfilled life. No forgiveness, no change: there is nothing in our lives that can be accomplished without forgiveness, reconciliation, pardoning, and self-acceptance.

Finally, changing fixed opinions and letting go of self-righteousness clear neurological pathways for us to reconnect with our selves. Pardoning someone for something they can't change is a decision that changes your life. Both paths of forgiveness can transform you into the man you have always wanted to be. This is what Eckhart Tolle refers to in his quote.

> *When you lose touch with your inner stillness, you lose touch with yourself. When you lose touch with yourself, you lose yourself in the world.*—Eckhart Tolle

Second Type of Forgiveness—You and Them

This second type of forgiveness is allowing the person who wronged you back in your life to have another chance. This is a courageous decision and a powerful act of self-love. Our ego can't let go of the wrongs committed but our core self can and chooses to do so. A loving approach to yourself is taking responsibility for your role in the situation. Considering your role in any conflict is freeing and empowering. If the person you allow back into your life chooses not to do so, that's his or her choice. The act of forgiving him or her is your choice. Putting aside the differences and weighing the value of this relationship is purposeful and productive.

What Happens to Me Now?
- Forgiveness is scary!
- Forgiveness is the ultimate act of courage and emotional maturity.

- Forgiveness breeds understanding, empathy, wisdom, responsibility, and peace of mind.
- Forgiveness is liberating for you.
- Forgiveness will change your life beyond expectation.

The positives of forgiveness far outweigh the ego's scorekeeping of personal wrongs. The personal benefit of releasing situations or people that you resent, are embarrassed about, or dislike is your mental health functioning at its best. All the psychological forefathers and foremothers agree that any type of reconciliation with yourself reaps tremendous benefits now and in your future.

Finally, forgiveness is not a one-and-done deal. It's not an emotional high but a calculated decision to let go and accept the situation as it is, not the way you want it to be. Accept the situation as it propels you forward from the tyranny of "why's" into a more compassionate perspective of you and your life.

Whatever the path you take to healing, forgiving, and resolving your childhood trauma, you might need to forgive some situations or people ten thousand times—and then one day it's done.

Men forgive; boys resent!

How Do I Forgive the Unforgiveable?

> *Healing doesn't mean the damage never existed. It means the damage no longer controls your life.*—Power of Positivity group

I recommend five steps to lessen your psychological load of personal injuries, resentments, and bitterness with peace of mind, emotional maturity, fulfilling relationships, and feeling content with your life. Forgiveness is a process, not a destination, achievement, or task.

Step 1—Acceptance

Accept the circumstances of the event, abuse, betrayal, incident, or person. This is challenging because you have to let go of what you think "should have been." It's imperative to accept that there is no "should" in life, only choices.

What is one of the most painful incidents or heartbreaks of your life that still bothers you?

Step 2—Hidden Lessons

What is the hidden value of this incident, the purpose for your personal growth, your personal awakening? Everything in your life has meaning; your responsibility is finding its buried meaning. There is value in our suffering, crying, depression, and losses. Look for the meaning separate from the emotional charge or anger surrounding it. There is something purposeful inside of this crisis. Let's consider the deeper meaning for you in the ashes of your life.

What is something I learned from this situation?

Step 3—Releasing Your Anger

What's the value of letting go of anger in my life? This is a tough challenge for men. We thrive on anger, but in the end, anger kills our heart, soul, and body. Releasing anger is an act of kindness, forgiveness, and a form of making amends with ourselves and the other person. This action requires us to stay connected to our adult emotional self without the need to retaliate or to feel sorry for ourselves. Letting go of our firewall of protection is a scary proposition. Unless you release your anger, you will never move forward in your life—nothing will change.

How is my anger protecting me?

Step 4—What Have I Learned about Relationships and Myself?

How can I handle things differently in my relationships in the future? How has this experience changed my perspective on relationships and my role in them? These questions illuminate the value of self-examination about our role in the disappointments of our lives. Learning about our needs and emotional blocks are all part of our healing process. Looking within to find the common patterns in our relationships helps us to make changes and create more stability for ourselves. There are patterns, needs, desires that appear in all your relationships.

What is something I have learned about myself in relationships?

Step 5—Leaving My Resentment in the Past

How has this incident or person helped me with redefining my life plans? It's impossible to move forward with one foot in the past and one foot in the present. You no longer replay, retell, or complain about the past incident. Your superpower is living in the present without looking backward. When you feel indifferent about the person, you have completed the process of forgiveness. The goal is indifference. A nonjudgmental emotional state is something that you can't buy, and it is yours for life. A reasonable goal for any disappointment, heartbreak, loss, professional setback is to learn, observe and release it.

> *The goal of forgiveness is becoming indifferent, no longer controlled by your past or the other person!*

What am I still holding on to from my past resentments?

MATURE MASCULINITY—WHAT DOES IT LOOK LIKE?

Choosing the way of a mature stand-up man there are certain masculine adult traits such as forgiveness. In chapter 13, we discussed the twelve common traits of immature men in a relationship. We now discuss twelve mature relationship qualities that enable us to forgive the unforgiveable.

Emotional maturity is the ability to access your feelings, understand the other person's position, and remain objective. These qualities are the positive side of masculinity; the immature qualities are the dark, unevolved, wounded side of a man. Forgiveness is the doorway to developing character qualities that all men want and that women want in their partners. There is a sense of safety, concern, and caring that comes from feeling understood and seen by your partner. Choosing to be kind rather than right in an argument creates an "energy bonus" that your partner carries inside of him or her. It's the picture that you create in your partner's heart of who and what you want to be to them and to yourself.

> *Women crave romantic partners with relationship skills who empower her life along with their own!*

The picture you carry inside of yourself will be the same one that your partner carries inside his or her heart. The twelve relationship ingredients are listed below. It's your challenge, responsibility, and reward to build these enduring qualities in yourself and in your relationship. They are the ingredients that make a man's life successful and prosperous.

Twelve Common Traits of Masculine Maturity

1. You are fully responsible for your actions, decisions, and the consequences of these choices. You don't start a sentence saying, "You made me feel and do this." Rather, you start the conversation, "I decided to do this."

2. You have a sense of who and what you are and how you behave in a relationship. You have individuated and have your own personality along with your four horsemen.
3. You are emotionally vulnerable with your partner about his or her struggles and concerns.
4. You accept feedback and constructive criticism about your actions and their impact on your partner and the family.
5. You tolerate differences of opinion and values. You are open-minded to suggestions and different perspectives.
6. You are emotionally stable, with predictable moods and behaviors. Your consistent behaviors form a secure bond between you and your partner.
7. You live in the present. You don't dwell in the past or argue about past issues.
8. You have a strong connection to your core self and to your values, priorities, and goals. You don't personalize other people's actions or disagreements as personal attacks.
9. You have emotional boundaries with yourself. You don't overshare personal information as a means of getting attention. You respect your partner's personal space and contributions to your life.
10. You approach difficult issues. You communicate in a positive way that engages your partner and his or her interests.
11. You are committed to the relationship and the ongoing work of building something special between the two of you. You accept that the things that happen in romantic relationships are part of the process and nothing to run from or avoid.
12. You prioritize your partner and the relationship. You enjoy being a couple, with or without children.

> *True masculinity is showing love, showing compassion, showing all these things that are traditionally not spoken of as masculine. And I think that scares some people.* —Keith Schmidt, Men's Project leader

PUTTING IT ALL TOGETHER—FIVE F-BOMBS FOR LIFE

Men have been bashed, overlooked, and rendered obsolete. Gentlemen have helped to create this state of affairs. We know it's time to be active participants in our lives and no longer wait to be invited to the party. Men are reconnecting to the brotherhood, recommitting to our responsibilities in five critical areas of our lives. These five areas are the true measurement of masculinity, brotherhood involvement, and who you are in your life.

It has taken us many chapters to build and finally put the universally approved blueprints of your life in your hands, heart, and mind. These five areas have been the cornerstones of every community, culture, and masculine journey.

Five "F-Bombs"

- *Family*—Responsibility to your past and present family members. You embrace your role in the family as a son, brother, husband.
- *Finances*—Supportive, responsible with money, career, work. You work and contribute to the well-being of your relationship. You "pay" your way through life.
- *Friends*—Fostering male bonds. We need male friends for support, advice, and accountability. Your partner isn't your only friend. Men can balance men. You develop or have a core support system of men.
- *Future*—Having a plan for your life—direction; purpose; and reason to get up in the morning—something to do and something to look forward to. You and your partner are walking forward with a shared life.
- *Forgiveness*—Men can't live without this ability to heal, to leave things in the past and to make emotional room for change. Your humility is a superpower and the result of being a forgiving man. You have developed courage, wisdom, and peace of mind by forgiving the unforgivable. Shame is powerless over you when confronted by your spirit and attitude of forgiveness.

Your Own Commencement Celebration

You have done it. You finally accessed the deepest, darkest part of your man cave. No one died from fear or emotional hunger. You have all the tools, wisdom, and practical knowledge to move forward on your individual journey. You truly "got this." You know what women want. You want to be the man you always wanted to be, even if no prior generations of men in your family ever became men whom you respected. You have a better understanding of your mental, physical, emotional, relational, and personal health. You accept that everything in your life is related and simultaneously separate. You have permission to symbolically leave home, love your family, create your own, build a career, mentor men and women, and empower the lost men in our lives.

Finally, your journey didn't start here and it's not ending here. You have the passion to go beyond the horizon of your limits and to see what's on the other side of that mountain. Many guys will quit but many men will not. Be that man who brings the brotherhood along. We will all benefit from your courageous life!

BIBLIOGRAPHY

Allen, Patricia, and Sandra Harmon. *Getting to "I Do": The Secret to Doing Relationships Right*. New York: Quill, 2002.

American Psychiatric Association. *Diagnostic and Statistical Manual of Mental Disorders*. 5th ed. Washington, DC: American Psychiatric Association, 2015.

Angelou, Maya. *Rainbow in the Cloud: The Wisdom and Spirit of Maya Angelou*. New York: New Press, 2014.

Beattie, Melody. *Codependent No More: How to Stop Controlling Others and Start Caring for Yourself*. Hazelden Foundation, 1987.

Bowen, Murray. *The Family Life Cycle*. New York: Gardner, 1988.

———. *The Use of Family Therapy in Clinical Practice*. Northvale, NJ: Jason Bronson Books, 1988.

Bowlby, John. *A Secure Base: Parent-Child Attachment and Healthy Human Development*. New York: Basic Books, 1988.

Bradshaw, John. *Homecoming: Reclaiming and Championing Your Inner Child*. New York: Bantam, 1990.

Brazen, T. Berry. *Working & Caring*. Reading, MA: Addison-Wesley, 1992.

Brown, Byron. *Soul without Shame: A Guide to Liberating Yourself from the Judge Within*. Boston: Shamble, 1999.

Bryan, Mark. *Codes of Love: How to Rethink Your Family and Remake Your Life*. New York: Pocket Books, 1999.

Chapman, Gary. *The Five Love Languages: How to Express Heartfelt Commitment to Your Mate*. Chicago: Northfield, 2004.

Dass, Ram. *Still Here: Embracing Aging, Changing and Dying*. New York: Riverhead, 2001.

Davis, Nadia. *Home is Within You—A Memoir of Recovery and Redemption*. Seattle: Girl Friday Books, 2023.

Dyer, Wayne W. *Wishes Fulfilled: Mastering the Art of Manifesting*. Carlsbad, CA: Hay House Publishers, 2012.

Goodpaster, Lisa. *Alienated—When Parents Won't Parent*. New York: Archway Publishing, 2023.

Hampel, John. *Wherever You Go, There You Are*. Milwaukee: Biff Publishers, 1991.

Hay, Louise L. *You Can Heal Your Life*. Santa Monica, CA: Hay House, 1987.

Insel, Thomas. *Healing—Our Path from Mental Illness to Mental Health*. New York: Penguin Random House, 2022.

Kubler-Ross, Elizabeth. *Working It Through: An Elizabeth Kubler-Ross Workshop on Life, Death and Transition*. New York: Simon & Schuster, 1997.

Mills, Jesse N. *A Field Guide to Men's Health—Eat Right, Stay Fit, Sleep Well, and Have Great Sex—Forever*. New York: Artisan, 2021.

Myss, Caroline M. *Defy Gravity: Healing beyond the Bounds of Reasons*. Carlsbad, CA: Hay House Publishers, 2009.

Parnell, Laurel. *A Therapist's Guide to EMDR—Tools and Techniques for Successful Treatment*. New York: W. W. Norton, 2007.

Peck, Scott M. *The Road Less Traveled: A New Psychology of Love, Traditional Values and Spiritual Growth*. 25th ed. New York: Touchstone Press, 2003.

Ruiz, Miguel. *The Four Agreements: A Personal Guide to Personal Freedom*. San Rafael, CA: Amber-Allen Publishers, 1997.

Schmidt, Gary D., and John Bunyan. *Pilgrim's Progress*. Grand Rapids, MI: W. B. Eerdmans Publishers, 1994.

Sogyal, Rinpoche. *The Tibetan Book of Living and Dying*. San Francisco: Harper Press, 1992.

Strong, Mary. *Letters of the Scattered Brotherhood*. New York: Harper Press, 1948.

Ullman, Dana. *Homeopathic Medicine for Children and Infants*. New York: Tarcher Perigee Press, 1992.

Van Der Kolf, Bessel. *The Body Keeps the Score—Brain, Mind and Body in the Healing of Trauma*. New York: Penguin Books, 2015.

Walsch, Neale Donald. *What God Said: The 25 Core Messages of Conversations with God That Will Change Your Life and World*. New York: Berkley Books, 2013.

Weil, Andrew. *Spontaneous Healing: How to Discover and Enhance Your Body's Natural Ability to Maintain and Heal Itself*. New York: Harper Press, 2006.

Yapko, Michael D. *Hand-Me-Down Blues—How to Stop Depression from Spreading in Families*. New York: St. Martin's Griffin, 1999.

Yogananda, Paramahansa. *Autobiography of a Yogi*. 13th ed. Los Angeles: International Publications of Self-Realization Fellowship, 2009.